Emergency Cross-S
Radiology

Emergency Cross-Sectional Radiology

Daniel Y. F. Chung
Speciality Registrar in Clinical Radiology, Oxford University Hospitals NHS Trust, Oxford, UK
Academic Clinical Fellow, Oxford University Clinical Academic Graduate School, Oxford, UK

Dipanjali Mondal
Speciality Registrar in Clinical Radiology, Oxford University Hospitals NHS Trust, Oxford, UK

Erskine J. Holmes
Emergency Medicine Consultant, Wexham Park Hospital, Slough, UK

Rakesh R. Misra
Consultant Radiologist, Wycombe Hospital, Buckinghamshire, UK

CAMBRIDGE
UNIVERSITY PRESS

CAMBRIDGE UNIVERSITY PRESS
Cambridge, New York, Melbourne, Madrid, Cape Town,
Singapore, São Paulo, Delhi, Tokyo, Mexico City

Cambridge University Press
The Edinburgh Building, Cambridge CB2 8RU, UK

Published in the United States of America by Cambridge University Press, New York

www.cambridge.org
Information on this title: www.cambridge.org/9780521279536

First published 2012

Printed in the United Kingdom at the University Press, Cambridge

A catalogue record for this publication is available from the British Library

Library of Congress Cataloguing in Publication data
Emergency cross-sectional radiology / Daniel Y.F. Chung ... [et al.].
   p.   ;   cm.
Includes bibliographical references and index.
ISBN 978-0-521-27953-6 (pbk.)
I. Chung, Daniel Y. F., 1982–
[DNLM: 1. Diagnostic Imaging – methods.   2. Anatomy, Cross-Sectional.
3. Critical Care – methods.   4. Emergencies.   5. Emergency Treatment – methods. WN 180]
LC classification not assigned
616.07'57–dc23

                                                                        2011031557

ISBN 978-0-521-27953-6 Paperback

I dedicate this book to my parents and my sister, Dona, for their continual support and sacrifices. **D. Y. C.**

To my dear parents, sister and brother, who have nurtured me from a young age. For their eternal guidance and support. **D. M.**

For my children, Alex and Amber, for the happiness they bring into our lives. **E. J. H.**

Dedicated to my beautiful wife Rachel, and children Rohan, Ela, Krishan and Maya, for allowing me the time to write this book. **R. R. M.**

Contents

Section 1   Fundamentals of cross-sectional imaging

Section 2   Pathology – Head and neck

Chest

Abdomen and pelvis

Abbreviations

AAA	Abdominal aortic aneurysm	FLAIR	Fluid-attenuated inversion recovery
AAST	American Association for the Surgery of Trauma	GCS	Glasgow coma scale
ABC	Airways, breathing, circulation	GI	Gastrointestinal
ACL	Anterior cruciate ligament	HII	Hypoxic-ischaemic injury
ACom	Anterior communicating	HIV	Human immunodeficiency virus
ADC	Apparent diffusion coefficient	HU	Hounsfield unit
AO	Aorta	ICA	Internal carotid artery
AP	Anteroposterior	i.m.	Intramuscular
APP	Appendicolith	IMA	Inferior mesenteric artery
ARDS	Acute respiratory distress syndrome	i.v.	Intravenous
AVM	Arteriovenous malformation	IVC	Inferior vena cava
AXR	Abdominal x-ray	JVP	Jugular venous pressure
BLD	Bladder	LA	Left atrium
B-mode	Brightness mode	LBO	Large-bowel obstruction
BP	Blood pressure	LK	Left kidney
bpm	Beats per minute	LP	Lumbar puncture
CBD	Common bile duct	LUQ	Left upper quadrant
COPD	Chronic obstructive pulmonary disease	LV	Left ventricle
CSF	Cerebrospinal fluid	MCA	Middle cerebral artery
CT	Computed tomography	MCL	Medial collateral ligament
CTPA	Computed tomography pulmonary angiogram	MHz	Megahertz
		M-mode	Modulation mode
CVA	Cerebrovascular accident	MRCP	Magnetic resonance cholangiopancreatography
CXR	Chest x-ray	MRI	Magnetic resonance imaging
DVT	Deep vein thrombosis	NF	Neurofibromatosis
DWI	Diffusion-weighted imaging	NIH	National Institutes of Health
ECA	External carotid artery	OMEN	Omentum
ECG	Electrocardiogram	PCL	Posterior cruciate ligament
eFAST	Extended focused assessment with sonography in trauma	PCom	Posterior communicating
		PCR	Polymerase chain reaction
ERCP	Endoscopic retrograde cholangiopancreatography	PD	Proton density
		PE	Pulmonary embolism
FAST	Focused assessment with sonography in trauma	PUJ	Pelvi-ureteric junction
		RA	Right atrium
		RF	Radio-frequency
Fat Sat	Fat saturation	RIF	Right iliac fossa

RK	Right kidney	TB	Tuberculosis
RUQ	Right upper quadrant	TE	Time to echo
RV	Right ventricle	TEMS	Transanal endoscopic microsurgery
SAH	Subarachnoid haemorrhage		
SBO	Small-bowel obstruction	TIA	Transient ischaemic attack
SDH	Subdural haemorrhage	t-PA	Tissue plasminogen activator
SMA	Superior mesenteric artery		
SPL	Spleen	TR	Time to repetition
STIR	Short tau inversion recovery	V/Q	Ventilation/perfusion scan
T1W	T1-weighted	VB	Vertebral body
T2W	T2-weighted	VUJ	Vesico-ureteric junction

Preface

Cross-sectional imaging – namely ultrasound, computed tomography and magnetic resonance imaging – is playing an ever more important role in the management of the acutely ill patient. There is a growing demand for radiologists at all levels of training to interpret complex studies and, alongside this, an increasing expectation that physicians should be able to recognize the important features of cross-sectional anatomy and pathology in order to expedite patient management.

Emergency Cross-Sectional Radiology aims to address both these expectations. Section 1 – 'Fundamentals of cross-sectional imaging' – aims to demystify cross-sectional imaging techniques for acute-care physicians who may be unfamiliar with the technical aspects of these modalities. Section 2 – 'Pathology' – describes a wide range of emergency conditions in an easy-to-read bullet-point format, with a large number of high-quality axial images used throughout. In addition, high-quality multiplanar reformats have also been included, where necessary, to illustrate and reinforce the findings, making this an invaluable rapid reference in everyday clinical practice. Recognizing the value of point-of-care ultrasound in the acute setting, a discussion of suitable applications and ultrasound findings has been included in the relevant chapters.

We hope that this book will be an invaluable practical aide-memoire for emergency-medicine physicians, surgeons, and acute-care physicians as well as radiologists in everyday reporting and in the emergency on-call environment to aid decision making.

Acknowledgements

Thank you to all the consultant radiologists in the Oxford Deanery, who have helped us throughout our training.

Dr Matthew Burn, Consultant Stroke Physician, Buckinghamshire Healthcare NHS Trust, edited the final manuscript and provided invaluable advice from a stroke physician's perspective. His contribution is greatly appreciated.

Dr Richard Hughes, Consultant Radiologist, Buckinghamshire Healthcare NHS Trust, provided several key images.

Sincere thanks to Luc Bouwman, CT Product Manager, Toshiba Medical Systems, Europe, for meticulously drawing all the superb images in Section 1: Fundamentals of cross-sectional imaging.

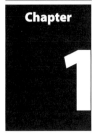

Chapter

Computed tomography

History

- In the early 1970s, Sir Godfrey Hounsfield's research team produced the first clinically useful computed tomography (CT) scans.

- The original scanners took approximately 6 minutes to perform a rotation (one slice) and 20 minutes to reconstruct it (Fig. 1.1a). Despite many technological advances since then, the principles remain the same.

- On early scanners, the tube rotated around a stationary patient, with the table moving to enable further acquisitions. The machine rotated clockwise and counter-clockwise as power was supplied via a cable.

- Modern-day helical or spiral scanners obtain power via slip ring technology, thus allowing continuous tube rotation as the patient moves through the scanner automatically (Fig. 1.1b). This allows a large amount of data to be acquired in a single rotation, with the benefits of faster scanning, faster patient throughput and fewer patient movement artefacts.

- New multi-slice scanners use existing helical scanning technology, but have multiple rows of detectors to acquire multiple slices per tube rotation. The faster imaging with multi-slice scanners allows a larger volume of coverage and multiphase scanning during intravenous contrast administration (Fig. 1.2). This, coupled with improved spatial resolution, allows organ-specific as well as peripheral vascular assessment, leading to the advent of CT angiography and virtual endoscopy.

- Advanced computer processing power allows reconstructive techniques, such as three-dimensional and multiplanar reformating, providing us with additional tools with which to improve diagnostic accuracy and aid clinical management.

Technical details

- The x-ray tube produces a narrow fan-shaped beam of collimated x-rays, which pass through the patient to reach a bank of detectors opposite the source (Fig. 1.3).

- X-rays are attenuated differentially by the patient, depending on the tissues through which they pass. Low-density tissues such as fat and aerated lung absorb fewer x-rays, allowing more to reach the detector. The opposite is true for dense tissues such as bone.

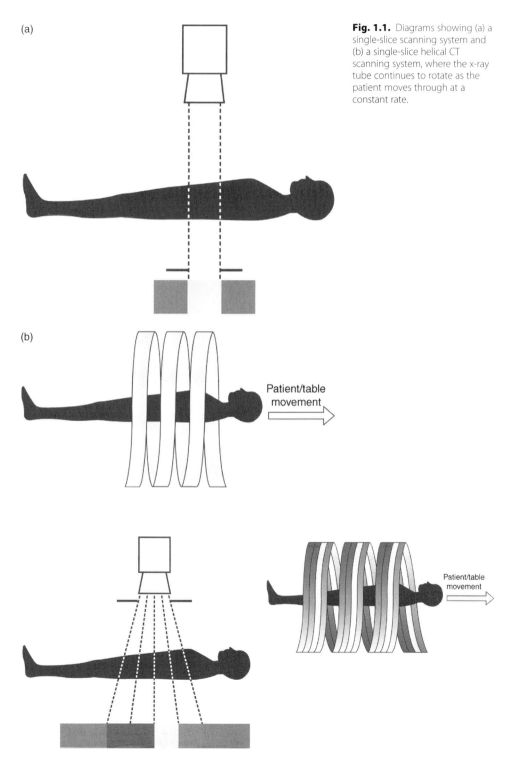

(a)

(b)

Fig. 1.1. Diagrams showing (a) a single-slice scanning system and (b) a single-slice helical CT scanning system, where the x-ray tube continues to rotate as the patient moves through at a constant rate.

Patient/table movement

Patient/table movement

Fig. 1.2. Multi-slice helical CT scanner with four detectors.

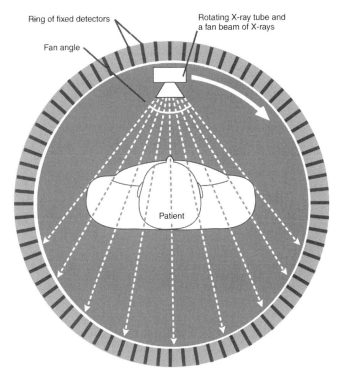

Ring of fixed detectors

Fan angle

Rotating X-ray tube and
a fan beam of X-rays

Patient

Fig. 1.3. Helical-ring system demonstrating the path of the x-rays from source to detector.

- The amount of transmitted x-ray radiation received by the detector provides information about the density of the tissue through which it has passed.
- A CT slice is divided up into a matrix of squares, e.g. 256×256, 512×512 and $1,024 \times 1,024$. The slice thickness determines the volume of these squares: these are called voxels. Using mathematical calculations, the degree to which a tissue absorbs radiation within each voxel, the *linear attenuation coefficient* μ, is calculated and assigned a value related to the average attenuation of the tissues within it – the *CT number* or *Hounsfield unit (HU)*.
- Each value of μ is assigned a greyscale value on the display monitor and is presented as a square picture element (pixel) on the image.
- Spiral scanners acquire a volume of information from which an axial slice is reconstructed, as above, using computer technology. Slices are created from the data during the reconstruction phase.
- *Pitch* is defined as the distance moved by the table (in millimetres) during one complete rotation of the x-ray tube, divided by the slice thickness in millimetres. In general, increasing pitch (increase in table speed with a fixed slice thickness) reduces the radiation dose to the patient (Fig. 1.4). This, in turn, reduces the amount of radiation reaching the detector for interpretation, with the net result of reduced image resolution. A compromise usually exists between limiting the patient's radiation dose and diagnostic image quality.

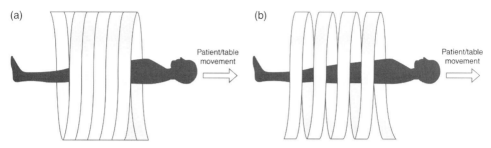

Fig. 1.4. Low pitch vs. high pitch: (a) low-pitch scanning with the table moving less for each tube revolution, resulting in a sharper image; (b) higher-pitch scanning, resulting in stretching of the helix as the table moves more for each revolution, leading to a loss of image quality.

Windowing and greyscale

- Modern CT scanners are able to differentiate in excess of 2,000 CT numbers; however, the human eye can only differentiate around 30 shades of grey.

- To maximize the perception of medically important features, images can be digitally processed to meet a variety of clinical requirements.

- The greyscale values assigned to process CT numbers on a display monitor can be adjusted to suit the requirements of particular applications.

- Contrast can be enhanced by assigning a narrow interval of CT numbers to the entire greyscale on the display monitor: this is called the *window technique*. The range of CT numbers displayed on the whole greyscale is called the *window width* and the average value is called the *window level*.

- Changes in window width alter contrast, and changes in window level select the structure of interest to be displayed on the greyscale, i.e. from black to white.

- Narrowing the window compresses the greyscale to enable better differentiation of tissues within the chosen window. For example, in the assessment of CT of the head, a narrow window of approximately 80 HU is used, with the centre at 30 HU. CT numbers above 70 (i.e. 30 + 40 HU) will appear white, and those below −10 (i.e. 30 − 40 HU) will appear black. This allows subtle differences in tissue densities to be identified.

- Conversely, if the window were widened to 1,500 HU, then each detectable shade of grey would cover 50 HU and soft-tissue differentiation would be lost; however, bone–soft tissue interfaces would be apparent.

- In practical terms, the window width and level are preset on the workstation and can be adjusted by choosing the appropriate setting, i.e. a window setting for brain, lung, bone, etc.

Tissue characteristics and contrast medium

- Unlike conventional radiography, CT has a relatively good contrast resolution and can therefore differentiate between tissues which vary only slightly in density (Fig. 1.5). This is extremely valuable when assessing the brain, as grey and white matter differ only slightly in density.

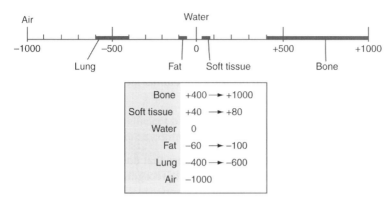

Fig. 1.5. Graphical representation showing Hounsfield scale and CT numbers for different types of tissue, water and air.

- In body CT, radio-opaque contrast agents are used to improve the quality of the study, depending on the clinical setting. This may be in the form of dilute barium (intraluminal contrast) or iodinated agents, which can be used both intravenously and intraluminally.

- Intravenous contrast agents opacify blood vessels, increasing the density of vascular abdominal organs, thereby improving the contrast between lesions and normal structures. Using multi-slice scanners, the passage of contrast through the arterial, parenchymal and venous systems can be assessed with multiphase imaging. On the other hand, intraluminal contrast agents distend the gastrointestinal tract to aid detection of luminal lesions.

- Intravenous contrast medium can also be used in both head and neck and body imaging to reveal abnormalities which are either vascular or disrupt the normal parenchyma. These can often be difficult to observe on an unenhanced study.

- The densest structure in the head is bone, which appears white on the CT scan. This is followed by acute haematoma, which is more dense than flowing blood due to clot retraction and loss of water. The hyperdensity of blood is due to the relative density of the haemoglobin molecule. Over time, blood appears isodense and then hypodense, compared with brain parenchyma due to clot resorption. The brain can be differentiated into grey and white matter due to the difference in fatty myelin content between the two. Typically, white matter (higher fatty myelin content: HU ≈ 30) is darker than the adjacent grey matter (HU ≈ 40).

- In body CT, bleeding sites are identified by focal areas of contrast medium extravasation, which appear as high-density linear streaks or blushes due to the relative high density of contrast medium. Alternatively, bleeding may also be indicated by increased density of intra-abdominal fluid (>50 HU) due to the mixing of blood or dense contrast medium with fluid of a density similar to that of water, i.e. <20 HU.

- Fat and air have low attenuation values, with a negative Hounsfield unit, and can readily be identified. Subtle pockets of air are best identified on lung windows, as will be demonstrated in later chapters. These are often difficult to appreciate in the abdomen against adjacent fat, which also appears dark.

Chapter

2

Magnetic resonance imaging

- Magnetic resonance imaging (MRI) is based on the principles of nuclear magnetic resonance (NMR), a spectroscopic technique used by scientists to study the chemical and physical properties of molecules at a microscopic level.

- In 1971, Raymond Damadian demonstrated that normal tissue and tumour tissue have different nuclear magnetic relaxation times. This raised the possibility of using magnetic resonance in clinical practice for disease detection.

- In 1977, the first MRI scan was performed on a human subject. It took almost 5 hours to produce one image.

- MRI is a rapidly developing imaging technique, which generates tomographic images safely and effectively.

- One of the major technological advantages of MRI is its ability to discriminate between different tissues according to their physical and biochemical properties. It therefore provides excellent soft-tissue contrast and is capable of demonstrating both anatomical features and flow-related phenomena. Unlike computed tomography (CT), MRI does not use ionizing radiation. Instead, it uses a powerful magnetic field to align the magnetization of some of the atoms in the body.

- The strength of a magnet in a MRI scanner ranges from 0.5 to 3 tesla (T), the unit of magnetic field strength. To put this into perspective, the Earth's magnetic field strength ranges from 0.00003 to 0.00007 T.

- In order to appreciate the complexities involved in image acquisition and interpretation of MRI, a basic understanding of MRI physics is required.

MRI physics

- MRI involves exploring the magnetic properties of human tissues. Hydrogen atoms, or protons, are essential components in human tissues; they provide the signal in MRI, which produces useful information.

- Hydrogen atoms are abundant in the human body, primarily in the form of water and fat. These protons have a single positive charge and spin on their own axis like the Earth. Additionally, protons also precess at a given frequency like a spinning top (Fig. 2.1) and this moving electric charge (i.e. an electric current) produces a magnetic field.

(a)   (b)

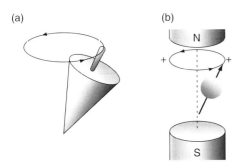

Fig. 2.1. (a) The motion of a spinning top describes how protons spin on their own axis and precess to produce a magnetic field. (b) Each proton possesses a positive charge. A moving charge (i.e. an electric current) induces a magnetic field.

- The human body can therefore be thought of as having millions of charged spinning protons, or bar magnets. Normally, these bar magnets are randomly aligned so that their charges cancel each other out, and thus there is no net magnetic moment.

- In an MRI scanner, an external magnetic field runs down the centre of the tube. When a patient is placed on the MRI table, the protons within the patient align themselves along the external magnetic field. The protons can either align with their north and south poles parallel to the external magnetic field or anti-parallel to it.

- These states have different energy levels, with the anti-parallel state requiring more energy. The desirable state is the one that requires the least amount of energy; that is, parallel to the external magnetic field.

- The difference between the two states is very small when placed in a magnet; the actual difference in the number of protons depends on the strength of the magnet. For every 10 million protons aligned anti-parallel to the magnetic field, approximately 10,000,007 will be aligned parallel to it. The majority of the protons therefore cancel each other out, leaving only a few unmatched protons per million, which result in a net longitudinal magnetic vector.

- The protons in the patient precess at a frequency that is proportional to the strength of the magnetic field. The equation that allows us to calculate this is known as the Larmor equation:

$$\omega_0 = \gamma B_0$$

where ω_0 = angular precession frequency in megahertz (MHz), γ = gyromagnetic ratio, and B_0 = external magnetic field in tesla (T).

- This means that as the external magnetic field strength increases, the precession frequency also increases. This relationship is determined by the gyromagnetic ratio (γ), which is different for different materials. For protons, this value is 42.5 MHz/T.

- Once the patient is placed into the magnet, a radio-frequency (RF) pulse is then applied to the patient through a coil. The RF pulse has the same frequency as that of the protons in the patient, known as the resonance frequency. There are two important effects of the RF pulse:

  - Some of the protons are elevated to a higher energy level (i.e. align anti-parallel to the magnetic field).

  - The protons are forced to precess in synchrony (in phase).

- The first effect causes the longitudinal magnetization to decrease, as there are now more protons aligned anti-parallel to the external magnetic field. The second effect creates a new magnetization called the transverse magnetization.
- Once the radio-frequency pulse is switched off, two major processes occur:
  - First, the protons that were raised to a higher energy level by the RF pulse now resume their original lower energy level, and in so doing release energy to the surrounding lattice. This is known as the longitudinal relaxation, spin-lattice relaxation or T1 relaxation. The protons point parallel to the magnetic field once more and thus the longitudinal magnetization increases, eventually going back to its original value. If this were to be graphically represented with time versus longitudinal magnetization, a characteristic curve is produced, known as the T1 curve (Fig. 2.2).
  - The second process to occur is that the protons no longer precess in synchrony, or in phase. The original external magnetic field is not completely homogeneous, resulting in protons with slightly different precession frequencies. Further to this, protons are influenced by the tiny magnetic fields of neighbouring protons, thus causing different precessing frequencies. By losing phase coherence, the protons start to point in different directions and therefore transverse magnetization decreases. This is known as transverse relaxation or T2 relaxation. By plotting time against transverse magnetization, a further characteristic curve is produced, known as the T2 curve (Fig. 2.3).
- Recovery of longitudinal relaxation and loss of transverse magnetization results in a change in direction of the magnetic moment which, in turn, induces an electric current

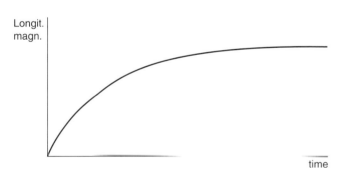

Fig. 2.2. T1 curve: graph plot of longitudinal magnetization vs. time after the RF pulse is switched off.

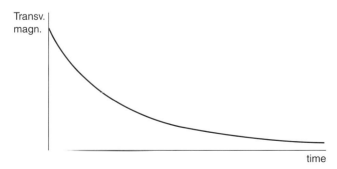

Fig. 2.3. T2 curve: graph plot of transverse magnetization vs. time after the RF pulse is switched off.

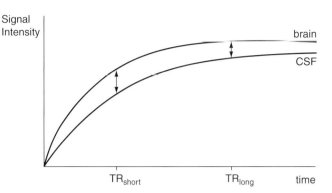

Signal Intensity

brain

CSF

TR_{short} TR_{long} time

Fig. 2.4. Graph demonstrating the shorter longitudinal relaxation time of brain vs. CSF. With a short time to repetition (TR), the signal intensities of brain and CSF differ more than after a long TR.

which is received by an antenna or detector coil. The signal produced is known as free induction decay (FID).

- The T1 and T2 curves are slightly different, depending on the tissue from which the signal comes. The rate of T1 and T2 relaxation is therefore tissue-dependent (i.e. fat or water) (Fig. 2.4).

- By sending sequential RF pulses, and varying the timing of signal sampling, useful information can be obtained about the tissues in question. In the above example, if a second RF pulse is sent within a short time interval – or time to repetition (TR) – then there will be a greater difference between the brain (fat) and cerebrospinal fluid (CSF, analogous with water) signal, and this will therefore give us the best tissue contrast.

- If the second RF pulse is sent in after a long TR, then the difference between the signal produced by the brain and CSF is very little and so the tissue contrast will be poor. The time between the RF pulse and the time when the signal is sampled is known as time to echo (TE).

- Standard sequences have been derived to differentiate one tissue from another. Three of the more common sequences are T1-weighted, T2-weighted and proton density. By looking at an image, one should be able to determine which sequence has been performed by the appearance of the different tissues, and also by identifying the parameters used. Detailed explanations of scanning parameters and more complex sequences is beyond the scope of this book; however, the following section briefly describes the most common sequences.

T1-weighted (T1W) (short TR (<500 ms), short TE (<50 ms)) (Fig. 2.5a)

- Exploits differences in T1 relaxation between tissues.
- Provides good anatomical detail.
- Fat is bright, as is protein, acute blood (<3 days old), melanin and contrast material (gadolinium).
- Water is dark.

T2-weighted (T2W) (long TR (>1,500 ms), long TE (>80 ms)) (Fig. 2.5b)

- Exploits differences in T2 relaxation between tissues.
- Sensitive in detecting oedema and therefore localizing pathology.

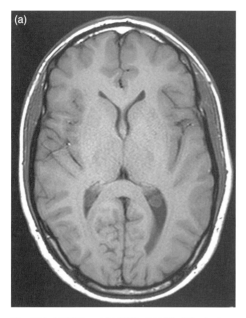 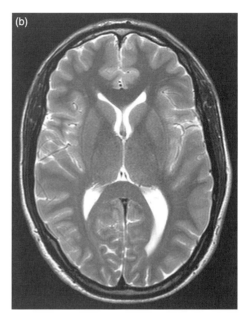

Fig. 2.5. (a) T1W and (b) T2W axial MRI of the brain.

- Fat is bright.
- Water is bright.

Proton density (PD) (long TR (>1,500 ms), short TE (<50 ms))

- Fat is bright.
- Water is dark.

	Grey matter	White matter	CSF
T1W (Fig. 2.5a)	Grey	White	Dark
T2W (Fig. 2.5b)	Grey	Dark	Bright
PD	Grey	Dark	Dark

- There are a few materials that are devoid of signal (black) on all sequences, due to their properties. Cortical bone and air are always black.

Contrast agents

- Contrast media such as gadolinium are used to enhance blood vessels and certain tissues.
- Gadolinium is a paramagnetic substance that has a small local magnetic field, which causes shortening of both the T1 and T2 relaxation times of surrounding protons. This has the effect of moving both the T1 and T2 curves to the left (Fig. 2.6).

(a)

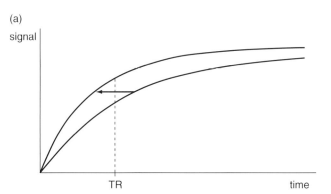

signal

TR   time

Fig. 2.6. Graphs demonstrating the effect of gadolinium, which shortens (a) T1 and (b) T2 relaxation times, shifting the curves to the left. At certain TR and TE values, the signal will be altered.

(b)

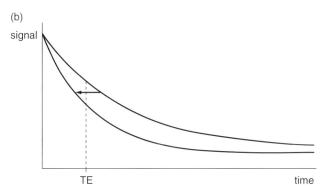

signal

TE   time

- The signal intensity increases on a T1-weighted image (Fig. 2.6a) and decreases on T2-weighted image (Fig. 2.6b). T1-weighted sequences are therefore preferred after contrast administration in order to provide better contrast.
- In its free state, gadolinium is toxic to humans, which is why it is bound to another chemical (DTPA) before being administered to patients.

Inversion recovery

- Inversion recovery sequences use a 180° RF pulse to invert the longitudinal magnetization vector to a negative value.
- As longitudinal magnetization recovers, it will eventually pass zero. This is known as the bounce point and is the point when the tissue will not generate an MRI signal. Thus tissue-specific time intervals (TI) are used before signal sampling to nullify the signal of certain tissues.

FLuid-Attenuated Inversion Recovery (FLAIR)

- This sequence uses a long TI, which corresponds to the bounce point of CSF (water).
- T2-weighted FLAIR images are often used in brain imaging to nullify the signal from CSF. In doing so, FLAIR sequences make periventricular and spinal cord lesions appear more conspicuous (Fig. 2.7).

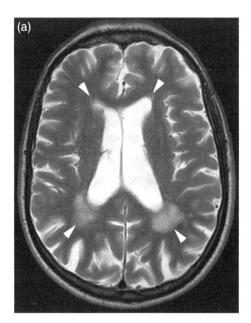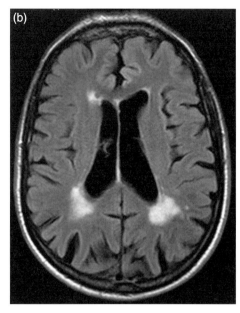

Fig. 2.7. Axial MRI of the brain. (a) T2W image demonstrating periventricular white matter high signal intensity consistent with small vessel ischaemic change (arrowheads). (b) FLAIR image demonstrating increased conspicuity of these changes when the high T2 CSF signal is nullified.

Short Tau Inversion Recovery (STIR)

- This sequence uses a shorter TI which corresponds to the bounce point of fat (bone marrow). STIR sequences are particularly useful in musculoskeletal imaging, where lesions and bone marrow oedema are accentuated by suppressing the signal from fat in bone marrow (Fig. 2.8).

Artefacts

- An image artefact is a positive or negative signal intensity within an image which does not actually represent the imaged anatomy. It is important to be aware of the following image artefacts.

Movement artefacts

- These artefacts are produced due to voluntary and involuntary movement (e.g. breathing) by the patient. Faint copies of the image are displaced vertically along the image to produce a 'ghost' image (Fig. 2.9).

Susceptibility artefacts

- Metallic objects within the body, such as a hip prosthesis or surgical clips, cause distortion of the local magnetic field, resulting in alteration/loss of signal in the surrounding tissues (Fig. 2.10).

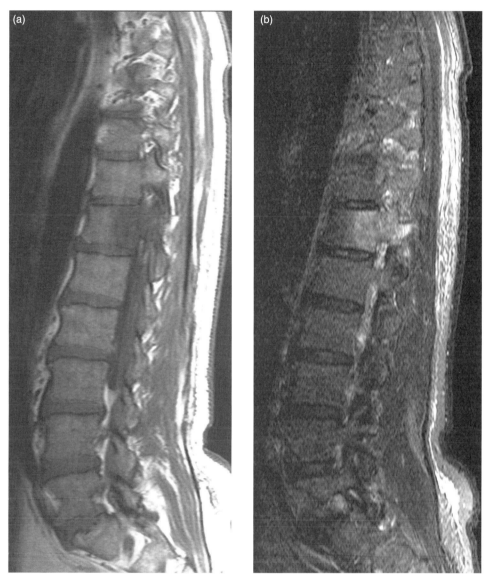

Fig. 2.8. Sagittal MRI of the lumbar spine. (a) T1W image demonstrating reduced bone marrow signal within the posterior T12 vertebral body, consistent with oedema secondary to osteomyelitis. (b) STIR images demonstrating increased conspicuity of the marrow oedema (high signal) after the high signal from marrow fat is suppressed in this sequence.

Chemical shift artefacts

- These occur due to the different chemical properties of fat and water, and are therefore artefacts seen at fat–water interfaces such as adjacent to abdominal organs.
- The artefact is seen as a dark band on the image in the horizontal direction.

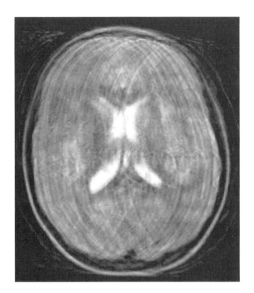

Fig. 2.9. Axial MRI of the brain demonstrating multiple 'ghost' images due to movement artefacts.

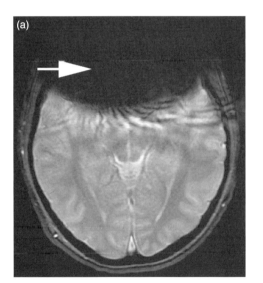

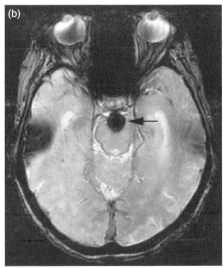

Fig. 2.10. Axial MRI of the brain demonstrating signal loss (arrow) secondary to (a) dental braces and (b) embolisation coils from previous cerebral aneurysm treatment, consistent with susceptibility artefacts.

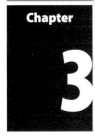

Chapter

3

Ultrasound

History

- Medical ultrasound has been established since the early 1940s. Commercially available systems were not widespread until the mid 1960s, and rapid technological advances have since expanded the scope of ultrasound significantly.

- Important progress has been made over the last decade in placing ultrasound machines at the patient's 'point of care', in the hands of experienced and trained clinicians who often have no formal radiological training. Formal ultrasound training and assessment systems are in place in the UK, and around the world, with recognition of core and enhanced skills acquisition and accreditation. There is now an acceptance of both diagnostic and procedural ultrasound outside radiology departments.

- Diagnostic ultrasound is deemed to be safe, without the disadvantages of ionizing radiation. With technical advances and new applications for use, safety aspects need to be continually reassessed.

- In the emergency-room setting, ultrasound is generally used to answer a specific focused question; e.g. is there blood within the peritoneal cavity in a trauma patient? Core competencies include eFAST (extended Focused Assessment with Sonography in Trauma), abdominal aortic aneurysm detection, ultrasound-guided line placement, and focused cardiac assessment. Procedural ultrasound guidance has been shown to reduce complication rates and improve success without a significant time delay.

- While it is accepted that CT is more sensitive and specific in the assessment of trauma, ultrasound also has a significant role to play.

Technical details

Piezoelectric effect

- Within the probe, there is an array of piezoelectric quartz crystals. When an electric current is applied to these crystals, they change shape rapidly, and this rapid shape change produces high-frequency sound waves (ultrasound) that travel outward.

- Ultrasound is defined as frequencies of >1 MHz. In clinical practice, frequencies between 2.5 and 15 MHz are used for medical imaging.

- Velocity or speed of ultrasound wave transmission is deemed to be constant for any given tissue. Transmission through soft tissues and fluids is good (1,540 m/s), **17** whereas it is poor through air (300 m/s). Ultrasound machines use the speed of propagation to calculate the depth of a structure, by measuring the time it takes for the sound wave to travel from the transducer to a structure and back again. The combination of depth, wave amplitude and orientation allows the machine to build and display an anatomical image.

Frequency vs. depth

- The higher the frequency, the greater the imaging resolution; however, frequency is inversely proportional to depth of imaging, due to tissue attenuation. Therefore, higher frequencies are appropriate for imaging superficial structures, and lower frequencies for deeper imaging. Most modern ultrasound machines allow frequency selection to be changed during a scan to optimize the displayed image.

Doppler imaging

- Movement within structures reflects the ultrasound signal, causing a frequency shift between the transmitted and received pulses (Doppler shift). Measurement of the magnitude of the Doppler shift allows velocity calculation, typically within blood vessels.

Duplex imaging

- Combines Doppler measurement with real-time imaging, allowing flow waveforms and anatomy to be simultaneously displayed.

Colour flow imaging

- Doppler information is displayed within the real-time image. Directional flow is colour coded, typically displayed as red or blue depending on the direction of flow.

Probe selection and scan technique

- Ultrasound probes differ in shape and scanning frequency, as follows:

LInear probes

- Emit a parallel beam (Fig. 3.1a), tend to be of higher frequency, and are generally used to image superficial structures and guide procedures, such as vascular access.

Curvilinear or sector probes

- Emit a divergent beam (Fig. 3.1b) and are usually of lower frequency, allowing wider and deeper tissue imaging.

- The probe face or 'footprint' is important and should be considered before scanning. Too large a footprint can limit scanning (e.g. between ribs), whereas a small footprint has a smaller field of view and is better suited to scanning smaller anatomical regions.

- Good scanning technique relies on choice of transducer, good contact between probe and skin, and a methodical well-practised procedure.

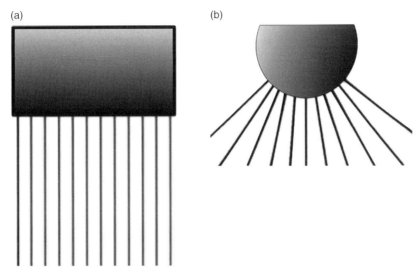

Fig. 3.1. Line drawings demonstrating (a) a parallel beam produced by a linear probe, and (b) a divergent beam emitted by a curvilinear probe.

Tissue characteristics and artefacts

- An ultrasound machine assumes that ultrasound travels in a straight line and at a constant velocity, and uses this information to build an anatomical image.
- The transducer sends a narrow beam of pulses and listens for reflections occurring at tissue interfaces. Some sound is reflected and some transmitted, allowing for further reflections from deeper structures.
- Soft tissues appear grey, with a typically grainy echotexture, fluid appears black (anechoic) and the surface of bone bright white, as all sound is reflected or absorbed, with no through transmission.

Posterior acoustic shadowing

- Occurs when a strongly reflective structure prevents the sound beam from travelling further into tissues, and therefore no echoes are produced from beyond this structure, e.g. gallstones and bone (Fig. 3.2a).

Posterior acoustic enhancement

- Produced when the sound beam passes through a structure that is less attenuating than the surrounding tissues, resulting in enhancement of echoes deep to the low-attenuating structure. Seen with free or contained fluid, e.g. bladder or cysts (Fig. 3.2b).

Reverberation

- Caused by the reflection of ultrasound waves between two highly reflective interfaces. Commonly seen at soft tissue–gas interfaces, e.g. pleural–air interface in thoracic imaging, and foreign body–soft tissue interfaces (Fig. 3.2c).

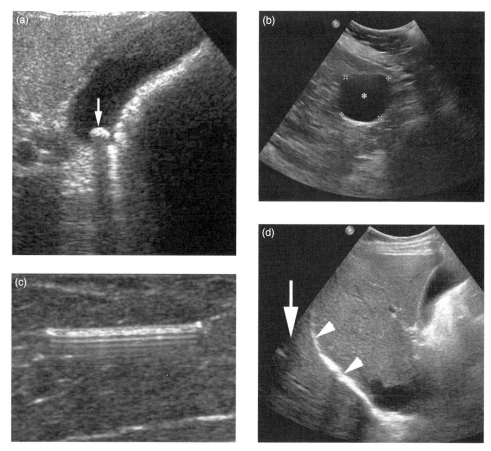

Fig. 3.2. Ultrasound images demonstrating artefacts. (a) Highly echogenic gallstone (arrow) prevents the passage of a sound wave, resulting in the absence of echo deep to the gallstone: termed *posterior acoustic shadowing*. (b) Anechoic cyst (asterix) does not attenuate the passage of the sound wave, resulting in enhancement of echoes deep to the cyst: *posterior acoustic enhancement*. (c) *Reverberation artefact* due to a metallic foreign body within the soft tissue. (d) The highly reflective pleural–air interface (arrowheads) creates the false impression of liver parenchyma deep to the diaphragm (arrow): *mirror-image artefact*.

Mirror-image artefact

- Occurs when an ultrasound wave encounters a highly reflective interface, resulting in the display showing a duplicated structure deep to this interface.
- This usually occurs at the level of the diaphragm, where the pleural–air interface acts as the highly reflective surface, with the effect that the liver parenchyma appears deep to the diaphragm (Fig. 3.2d).

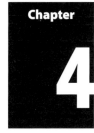

Chapter

4

Acute stroke

Characteristics

- Stroke is the third most common cause of death in the UK. In England alone, 110,000 people have a stroke every year. Stroke is the leading cause of adult disability, with >300,000 people in England living with moderate to severe disability as a result of stroke.

- Strokes are broadly divided into two groups: ischaemic and haemorrhagic. Ischaemic strokes are caused by thrombosis or embolism, and are more common than haemorrhagic strokes.

- Haemorrhagic strokes account for 15% of all strokes, usually caused by hypertensive damage to small intracerebral arteries, causing rupture and leakage of blood directly into the parenchyma. This results in surrounding oedema and mass effect, further compromising the adjacent blood supply.

- Transient ischaemic attack (TIA) is defined as a neurological deficit that resolves within 24 hours. About 10–15% of patients who have had a TIA suffer a stroke within 90 days – half of them within the first few days. The risk is highest in those patients with carotid artery stenosis or atrial fibrillation. The *ABCD^2 score* (see Appendix I) is widely used in clinical practice to divide patients into risk categories for further investigation and treatment.

- The incidence of stroke increases with age, although one-quarter occur in the under-65s.

- Risk factors include hypertension, smoking, diabetes, heart disease (coronary artery disease, cardiomyopathy, chronic atrial fibrillation), hyperlipidaemia, atherosclerosis, the oral contraceptive pill and obesity. Underlying brain pathology (e.g. tumour), a predisposition to bleeding (bleeding diathesis), anticoagulation treatment and thrombolysis therapy are additional risk factors specific to haemorrhagic strokes. Cocaine use is a risk factor for both ischaemic and haemorrhagic strokes.

- Thrombolysis therapy has been shown by the National Institute of Neurologic Disorders and Stroke (NINDS) t-PA Pilot Trial to have a positive effect, if tissue plasminogen activator (t-PA) is administered within a 3-hour window, for a patient deemed likely to benefit from thrombolytic intervention. This treatment window is likely to become wider, based on the European Cooperative Acute Stroke Study III (ECASS III), demonstrating efficacy in improving neurologic outcomes following the use of thrombolytic therapy between 3 and 4.5 hours after the onset of symptoms. Timely access to brain imaging will play an increasingly vital role in the provision of an effective thrombolysis service.

Clinical features

- Haemorrhagic and ischaemic strokes are difficult to distinguish clinically, and the only reliable way to differentiate between them is by using brain imaging. The spectrum of presentation can range from mild symptoms and signs in a healthy patient, to a moribund comatosed condition.

- Patients with haemorrhagic strokes tend to be more unwell, with abrupt symptom onset and rapid deterioration. Common symptoms include headache, decreased consciousness level, seizures, nausea and vomiting. Hypertension is characteristic.

- Ischaemic strokes have a varied presentation depending on the vascular territory involved, commonly presenting with unilateral weakness and/or sensory loss, visual field defect, aphasia and inattention/neglect.

- Deep white matter infarcts (lacunar infarcts) typically present with a pure motor and/or sensory deficit with an absence of features suggesting cortical involvement (visual field defect, aphasia or inattention/neglect). Posterior circulation infarcts commonly present with vertigo, ataxia, diplopia, dysarthria or dysphagia, and sometimes with bilateral limb signs due to brainstem involvement.

- The neurological deficit can be sudden and often occurs during sleep, making the time of onset difficult to ascertain.

Radiological features

CT

- Aims to identify any contraindication to thrombolysis rather than confirming the diagnosis.

- Contraindications include:.
  - Haemorrhage
  - More than one-third of middle cerebral artery (MCA) territory involvement (i.e. an increased risk of haemorrhage with thrombolysis and therefore a relative contraindication).

- Using the 10-point ASPECTS (Alberta Stroke Program Early CT Score) system ensures systematic interpretation of brain CT, and is useful in determining prognosis.

Features
Ischaemic stroke

Hyperacute infarction (<12 hours)

- Non-contrast CT may appear normal in up to 60% of cases.

- Contrary to general opinion, the CT may be abnormal in up to 75% of patients with MCA infarction imaged within the first 3 hours.

- *Hyperdense vessel sign* represents acute intraluminal thrombus, recognized as focal or linear increased (white) density within the artery on a non-contrast CT of the head. This is most commonly seen in MCA occlusion, in 25–50% of cases (Fig. 4.1), although it can be present in other intracranial arteries.

- *Lentiform sign* denotes obscuration of the normally well-defined lentiform nucleus, occurring in 50 80% of acute MCA occlusions (Fig. 4.2a).
- *Insular ribbon sign* describes the loss of grey–white matter differentiation in the lateral margins of the insular cortex, supplied by the insular segment of the MCA (Fig. 4.2b, c).

Acute infarction
   12–24 hours (Fig. 4.3a)

- Low-density basal ganglia.
- Loss of normal grey–white matter differentiation secondary to oedema.
- Loss of the normal sulcal pattern may indicate underlying oedema.

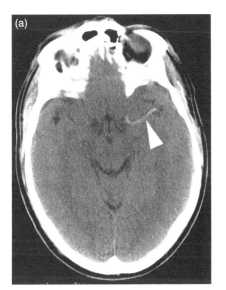
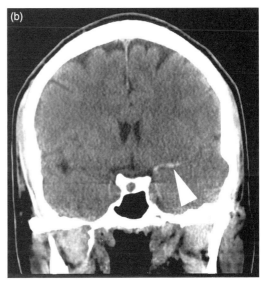

Fig. 4.1. (a) Axial and (b) coronal images demonstrating a hyperdense left MCA in keeping with acute intraluminal thrombus (arrowhead).

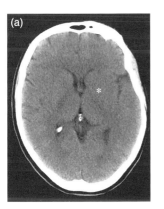
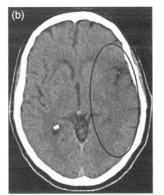
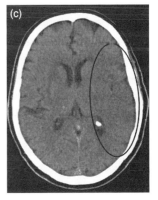

Fig. 4.2. (a) Axial image demonstrating subtle obscuration of the left lentiform nucleus (asterix), which is normally well defined, as seen on the contralateral side: the *lentiform sign*. (b), (c) Axial images demonstrating subtle loss of grey–white matter differentiation at the lateral margin of the insular cortex: the *insular ribbon sign*.

1–7 days (Figs. 4.3b and 4.4)

- Area of hypodensity in a vascular distribution (in 70% of cases) due to cytotoxic oedema.
- Mass effect secondary to oedema, resulting in local or generalized compression of the ventricles, basal cisterns and midline shift.
- Haemorrhagic transformation may occur after 2–4 days in up to 70% of patients.

Subacute/chronic infarction (>7 days – months) (Fig. 4.5)

- Decrease in mass effect and ex-vacuo dilatation of the ventricles to occupy the potential space resulting from infarcted brain parenchyma.
- Loss of parenchymal mass, with associated sulcal/ventricular widening, due to encephalomalacia.

Haemorrhagic stroke

- Non-contrast head CT is the investigation of choice, as contrast may obscure haematoma, which also appears dense on CT.
- Acute haemorrhage is hyperdense (Figs. 4.6 and 4.7).
- Surrounding oedema will result in loss of grey–white matter differentiation.
- Mass effect will result in compression of overlying sulci, ventricular compression, midline shift and reduction in the size of the basal cisterns.
- Site and size of the haemorrhage are important, and will influence future treatment options.

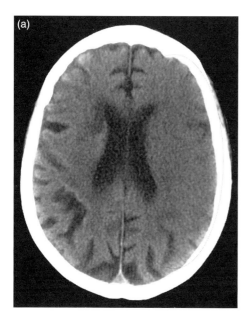 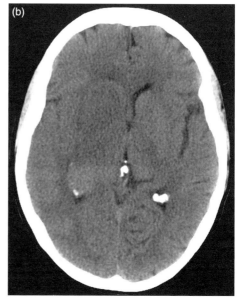

Fig. 4.3. (a) Early large left MCA infarct: axial image showing loss of grey–white matter differentiation and sulcal effacement secondary to oedema in the left MCA territory. (b) Early large right MCA infarct: obscuration of the right lentiform nucleus with low-attenuation oedema causing mass effect, compressing the right lateral ventricle.

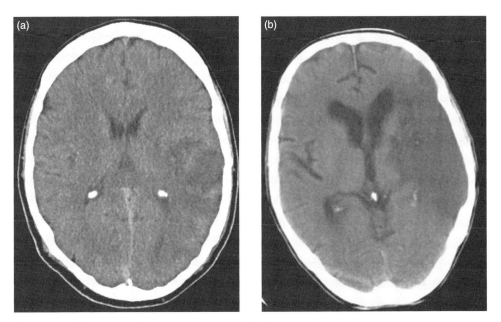

Fig. 4.4. (a), (b) Large areas of hypodensity within the left MCA territory due to cytotoxic oedema.

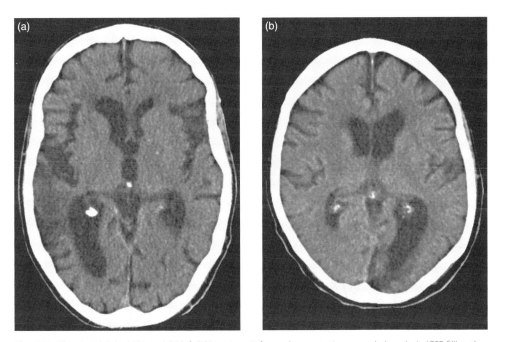

Fig. 4.5. Chronic (a) right MCA and (b) left PCA territory infarcts, demonstrating encephalomalacia (CSF filling the 'dead' space following infarction) and ex-vacuo dilatation of the adjacent ventricle.

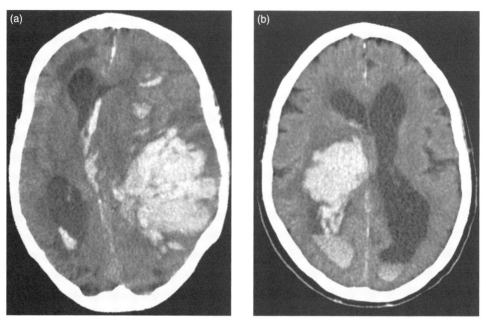

Fig. 4.6. (a) Large intracerebral haemorrhage within the left MCA territory, with rupture into the ventricular system. There is significant mass effect, with shift of midline structures to the right, and compression of the ipsilateral ventricle. (b) Acute haemorrhage centred on the right thalamus and lentiform nucleus with intraventricular rupture.

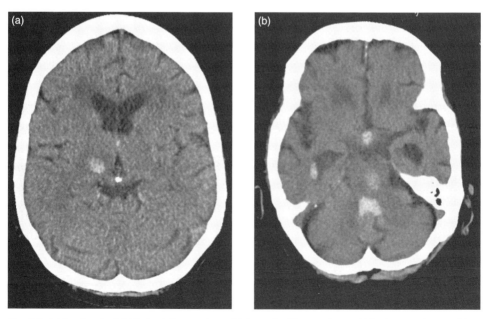

Fig. 4.7. (a) Small acute right thalamic haemorrhage. (b) Acute focal haemorrhage within the central pons with intraventricular extension.

MRI

Features

- Though not widely available in many centres, this technique benefits from not using ionizing radiation and has greater sensitivity and specificity than CT in the detection of cerebral ischaemia in the first few hours post insult.
- Specific features:
  - Hyperintense signal on T2/FLAIR (fluid-attenuated inversion recovery)
  - Sulcal effacement secondary to mass effect from cytotoxic oedema
  - Loss of arterial flow voids on T2/FLAIR and stasis of contrast material in vessels, secondary to reduced flow from intra-arterial thrombosis
  - Gradient echo imaging is sensitive to susceptibility artefacts, allowing haemorrhage to be detected (Fig. 4.8).
- Diffusion-weighted imaging (DWI) is particularly sensitive in hyperacute stroke assessment, with restricted diffusion observed as early as 30 minutes after the onset of stroke (Figs. 4.9 and 4.10). DWI also allows temporal evaluation of infarcts (see Table 4.1).

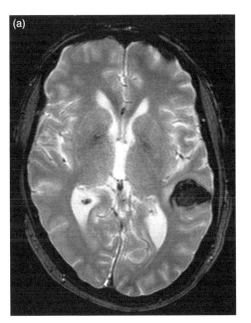 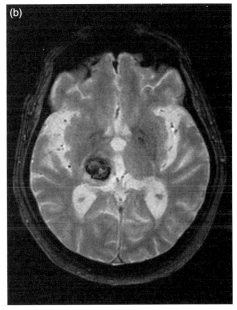

Fig. 4.8. T2* gradient echo MR images demonstrating susceptibility artefacts from intraparenchymal haemorrhage in (a) the left temporoparietal region and (b) the right thalamus.

Table 4.1 Temporal evaluation of infarcts using diffuse imaging (DWI, diffusion-weighted imaging, ADC, apparent diffusion coefficient).

	Hyperacute	Acute	Subacute	Chronic
DWI	Hyperintense	Hyperintense	Iso/Hyperintense	Variable
ADC	Hypointense	Hypointense	Iso/Hyperintense	Hyperintense

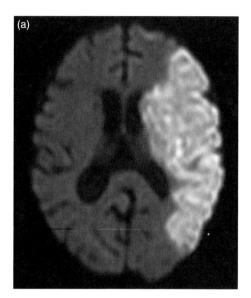
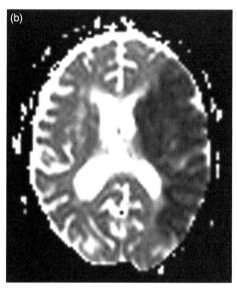

Fig. 4.9. Diffusion MR imaging: high signal intensity (restricted diffusion) on (a) DWI in the left middle cerebral artery territory with corresponding low signal intensity on (b) ADC, consistent with a hyperacute infarct.

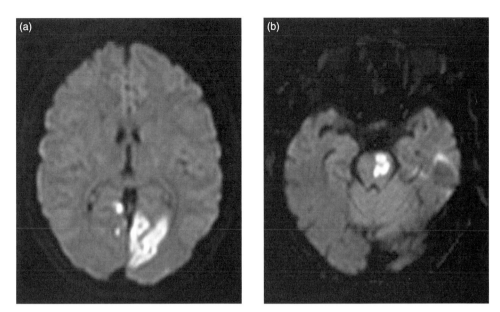

Fig. 4.10. DWI images demonstrating high signal restricted diffusion in (a) the left posterior cerebral artery territory and (b) the left pons, both of which demonstrate corresponding low signal intensity on ADC (not shown), consistent with hyperacute infarcts.

Chapter

5

Subdural haematoma

Characteristics

- Subdural haemorrhage arises between the dura and arachnoid membrane of the brain.
- Bleeding results from torn bridging veins that cross the potential space between the cerebral cortex and dural venous sinuses.
- Usually categorized into acute, subacute or chronic.
- Acute subdural haematoma (SDH) carries a high risk of mortality and morbidity, as it is more commonly associated with extensive primary brain injury. Direct pressure results in ischaemia on the adjacent brain tissue.
- Re-bleeding secondary to osmotic expansion, or further trauma, leads to acute-on-chronic haemorrhage.
- All causes of brain tissue loss (e.g. hydrocephalus and stroke) are considered risk factors. Elderly and alcohol-dependent patients' risks are often compounded by instability of gait and co-morbidity.
- The aetiology of chronic SDH is often unclear, although most likely from minor trauma in the preceding few weeks. In 50% of cases, no such history is obtainable.
- Subdural haemorrhage in the newborn is usually due to obstetric trauma. In paediatric patients, non-accidental injury needs to be considered.

Clinical features

Acute SDH

- Patients often present following severe head trauma, 50% associated with underlying brain injury, with a worse long-term prognosis than extradural haematoma.
- Patients generally have a decreased level of consciousness, with focal neurological defects or seizures. There may be signs of raised intracranial pressure.
- Patients with a primary or secondary coagulopathy (e.g. alcoholics, those undergoing anticoagulation therapy) may develop an acute SDH after only minor head trauma.
- A small acute SDH may be asymptomatic.

Chronic SDH

- Chronic SDH is the result of:
  - Resolving phase of medically managed acute subdural haematoma
  - Repeated episodes of subclinical haemorrhage, later becoming symptomatic.

- Chronic SDH often presents in the elderly with vague symptoms of gradual depression, personality change, fluctuation of consciousness, unexplained headaches, or evolving hemiplegia. Over 75% of cases occur in patients >50 years of age.

Radiological features

CT

- CT scan without contrast, as high-density contrast may obscure visualization of blood.

Location

- Blood is seen over the cerebral convexity, often extending into the interhemispheric fissure, along the tentorial margins, and beneath the temporal and occipital lobes (Fig. 5.1).
- Does not cross the midline, as it is limited by the falx cerebri.
- Bilateral in 15–25% of adults (most commonly in the elderly) and in 80–85% of infants.

Features
Acute SDH (<72 hours) (Fig. 5.2)

- Peripheral high-density crescentic fluid collection between the skull and cerebral hemisphere usually with:
  - A concave inner margin: a small haematoma may only minimally displace brain substance
  - Convex outer margin following normal contour of cranial vault
  - Occasionally, a blood-fluid level is seen secondary to high- and low-density fluid separation
  - Signs of mass effect with compression of overlying sulci, ventricular compression, midline shift and reduction in the size of the basal cisterns.

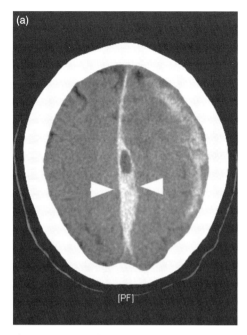
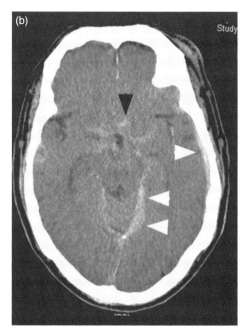

Fig. 5.1. Acute subdural haematoma on axial images (a) over the left cerebral convexity with additional acute-on-chronic haematoma extending along the interhemispheric fissure (arrowheads); (b) along the tentorium and over the left temporal lobe (white arrowheads). Additional subarachnoid haemorrhage is also present (black arrowhead).

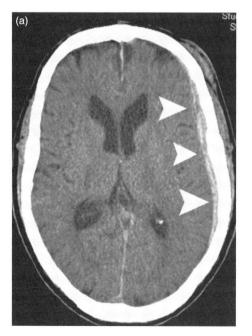
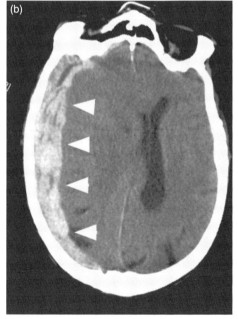

Fig. 5.2. Axial images showing (a) acute shallow left subdural haematoma (arrows), (b) large acute right subdural haematoma (arrowheads).

Subacute SDH (3–21 days) (Fig. 5.3)

- After approximately 1–2 weeks, the subdural collection becomes isodense to grey matter. Detection may be challenging and may only be recognized due to persistent mass effect:
  - Effacement of cortical sulci
  - Deviation of lateral ventricle
  - Midline shift, white-matter buckling
  - Displacement of grey–white matter interfaces.
- On contrast-enhanced CT scans, the cortical–subdural interface will be defined, with enhancement of the cerebral cortex and non-enhancement of the overlying haematoma.

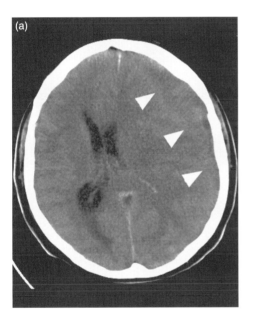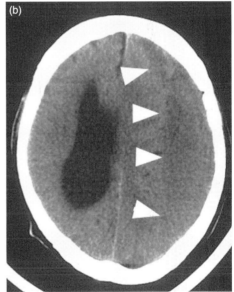

Fig. 5.3. Axial images showing (a) left isodense/hypodense subdural collection (arrowheads) with midline shift to the right; (b) large isodense subdural haematoma (arrowheads) with associated mass effect, compressing the left lateral ventricle and dilatation of the right lateral ventricle.

Chronic SDH (>21 days) (Fig. 5.4)

- These are often hypodense crescentic collections, with or without mass effect.
- Acute-on-chronic SDHs can further complicate the imaging, with hyperdense fresh haemorrhage intermixed, or layering posteriorly, within the chronic collection.
- Complex septated collections, and in rare cases calcification, may develop.

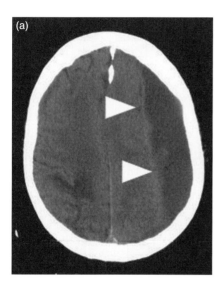 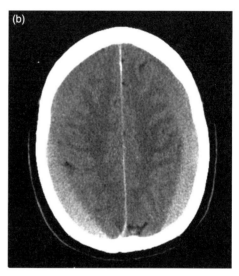

Fig. 5.4. Axial images showing (a) large left chronic subdural haematoma (arrowhead); (b) bilateral chronic subdural haematomas.

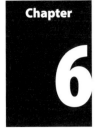

Chapter

6

Extradural/epidural haematoma

Characteristics

- Extra-axial haemorrhage arising within the potential space between the skull and dura mater.

- The dura becomes more adherent with age. The young are more frequently affected, as the dura is more easily stripped away from the skull.

- Associated with a skull fracture in 75–95% of cases.

- Occurs in 2% of all serious head injuries, though seen in <1% of all children with cranial trauma, as calvarial plasticity means that skull fractures are less common. In rare cases, extradural haematomas can occur spontaneously.

- Bleeding is commonly from a lacerated (middle) meningeal artery/vein, adjacent to the inner skull table, from a fracture crossing the path of the artery or dural branches.

- Early diagnosis is imperative, as prognosis is good with early intervention prior to neurological deterioration from cerebral herniation and brainstem compression.

- Types:
  - Acute extradural haematoma (60%) from arterial bleeding.
  - Subacute extradural haematoma (30%).
  - Chronic extradural haematoma (10%) from venous bleeding or a torn dural sinus (more common with posterior skull fractures).

Clinical features

- Patients often present with a history of head trauma associated with a variable level of consciousness.

- The classical 'talk and die' presentation, where a brief loss of consciousness occurs at the time of impact, followed by rapid neurological deterioration as the haematoma expands, only occurs in 20–50% of patients. Other symptoms may include headache, vomiting and seizures following head injury.

- Neurological examination may reveal lateralizing signs, with a unilateral up-going plantar reflex.

- A sensitive sign in the conscious patient is pronator drift of the upper limb.

- Close neurological observation is necessary to detect any alteration in consciousness, with changes in *Glasgow coma scale* (GCS) (see Appendix III) and rising intracranial pressure: clinically manifest as dilated, sluggish or fixed pupils, decerebrate posture, or Cushing response (hypertension, bradycardia and bradypnoea).

Radiological features

CT

- CT scan without contrast, as high-density contrast may obscure visualization of blood.

Location

- 66% temporoparietal (most often from laceration of the middle meningeal artery).
- 29% frontal pole, parieto-occipital region, between occipital lobes and posterior fossa (most often from laceration of the dural sinuses from a fracture).
- Disruption of the sagittal sinus may create a vertex epidural haematoma.

Features

- Biconvex hyperdense elliptical collection with a sharply defined edge (Fig. 6.1).
- Mixed high and low density suggests active bleeding, giving a 'whorled' appearance to the haematoma.
- Haematoma does not cross suture lines unless a diastatic suture fracture is present.
- Crosses dural reflections. May separate the venous sinuses and falx from the skull; this is the only type of intracranial haemorrhage to do this.
- Signs of mass effect such as sulcal effacement, ventricular compression, subfalcine herniation, effacement of the basal cisterns and tonsillar herniation may be present.
- Venous bleeding is more variable in shape.
- The study should be carefully scrutinized on bone windows due to the frequent association of skull fractures and extradural haematomas.

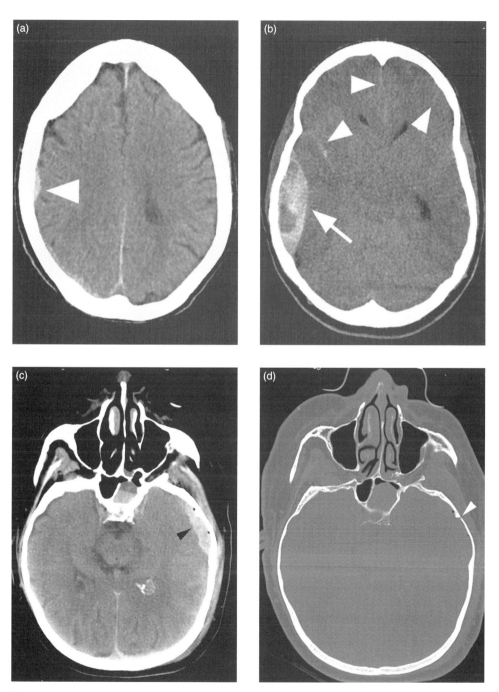

Fig. 6.1. Axial images demonstrating (a) subtle right acute extradural haemorrhage (arrowhead); (b) mixed-density right extradural haemorrhage indicating acute and subacute components (arrow). Note additional subarachnoid haemorrhage (arrowheads); (c) left extradural haemorrhage (black arrowhead) with low-attenuation gas locules secondary to an underlying skull fracture identified on (d) bone windows (white arrowhead). There is also high-attenuation blood within the left sphenoid sinus.

Chapter

7

Subarachnoid haemorrhage

Characteristics

- Subarachnoid haemorrhage (SAH) accounts for 6–8% of cerebrovascular accidents (CVAs). Recognized as a particularly important cause in younger patients. Its incidence remains constant despite other causes of CVAs showing a decrease.

- Causes:
    - Spontaneous – ruptured aneurysm (72%), arteriovenous malformation (AVM) (10%) and hypertensive haemorrhage.
    - Trauma.

- Blood enters the subarachnoid space between the pia and arachnoid mater which may lead to raised intracranial pressure by obstructing the ventricular outflow of CSF.

- Incidence increases with age and peaks at age 50 years. Approximately 80% of cases of SAH occur in people aged 40–65 years, with 15% occurring in people aged 20–40 years.

- 40–50% of patients with aneurysmal SAH have symptoms from a 'sentinel bleed' consistent with a small leak. This may occur a few hours to a few months before the rupture, with a median time of 2 weeks prior to diagnosis.

- An estimated 10–15% of patients die before reaching hospital and the mortality rate approaches 40% within the first week due to re-bleeding.

- Advances in management have resulted in reduced mortality, although more than one-third of survivors have major residual neurological deficits leading to long-term morbidity.

Clinical features

- SAH classically presents with a sudden onset of a severe 'thunderclap' headache, often described as the 'worst headache in my life'.

- Meningeal irritation generates symptoms of neck stiffness, photophobia and low back pain, with a positive Kernig's sign.

- 10–25% of patients develop seizures within minutes of the onset.

- Rise in intracranial pressure can lead to nausea and vomiting.

- Prodromal symptoms may also be reported and are not necessarily related to a 'sentinel bleed'.

- Focal neurological signs:

  ○ Oculomotor nerve palsy – compression by an expanding berry aneurysm of the posterior communicating artery of the circle of Willis.

  ○ Abducens nerve palsy – associated with increased intracranial pressure.

  ○ Mono-ocular visual loss due to ophthalmic artery aneurysm.

  ○ Unilateral leg weakness or paraparesis suggests anterior communicating artery aneurysm rupture.

- Fundoscopy may reveal papilloedema and subhyaloid retinal haemorrhages.

- Lumbar puncture (LP) is performed 12 hours after the onset of symptoms to evaluate for xanthochromia if the initial CT is negative for SAH. 15% of LPs are false negatives.

Radiological features

CT

- CT scan without contrast, as high-density contrast may obscure visualization of blood.

Location of aneurysm rupture

- Approximately 85% of saccular aneurysms occur in the anterior circulation. The most common sites of rupture are as follows:

  ○ The internal carotid artery, including the posterior communicating (PCom) artery junction (41%).

  ○ The anterior communicating (ACom) artery/anterior cerebral artery (34%)

  ○ The middle cerebral artery (MCA) (20%).

  ○ The vertebrobasilar and other arteries (5%).

Features

- CT scan findings are positive in approximately 92% of patients who have SAH.

- Sensitivity decreases with time; 98% within the first 12 hours and 93% within 24 hours. This decreases to 80% at 72 hours and 50% at 1 week.

- May be falsely negative in patients with small haemorrhages and in those with severe anaemia.

- The aneurysm may be apparent as a round soft-tissue density structure with or without rim calcification (Fig. 7.1)

- The location of blood within the subarachnoid space correlates directly with the location of the aneurysm rupture in 70% of cases:

  ○ Internal carotid artery – 4th ventricle, basal cistern and around brainstem.

  ○ ACom artery – interhemispheric and frontal horn intraventricular blood (Fig. 7.2a).

  ○ MCA – sylvian fissure and temporal lobe haematoma (Fig. 7.3a).

  ○ Vertebrobasilar arteries – interpeduncular or cerebellopontine angle cistern (Fig. 7.2b).

  ○ Blood found lying over the cerebral convexities or within the superficial brain parenchyma suggests rupture of an AVM or mycotic aneurysm.

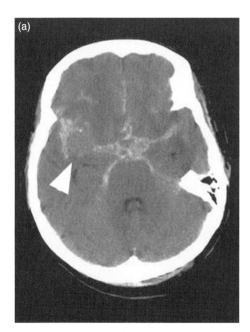 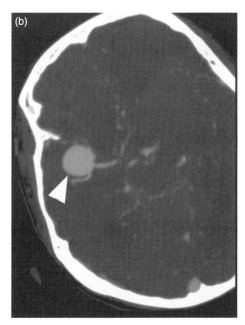

Fig. 7.1. (a) Axial image demonstrating extensive hyperdense subarachnoid blood within the basal cisterns secondary to a ruptured right MCA aneurysm (arrowhead); (b) CT angiogram showing large right MCA aneurysm (arrowhead).

- Mass effect: hydrocephalus and subfalcine/transtentorial herniation. This is due to reduced outflow/resorption of CSF by arachnoid granulations secondary to the haemorrhage, and may be present in up to 20% of patients.

- Subtle areas for review: high density within sulci, occipital horn of the lateral ventricles (blood/fluid level), interpeduncular cistern, and asymmetrical density of the tentorium cerebelli.

- A contrast-enhanced CT scan may reveal an underlying AVM; however, a non-contrast study should always be performed first.

CT angiography

Features

- There is continuing debate regarding its sensitivity compared with the gold standard of catheter angiography. It has the advantage of being non-invasive, reducing the small but important neurological risks related to conventional catheter angiography.

- Recent meta-analysis shows a sensitivity of 57–100% compared with conventional angiography and surgical findings, with higher sensitivity observed with newer multi-slice scanners. The most commonly missed aneurysms are those <4 mm in size and adjacent to the skull base.

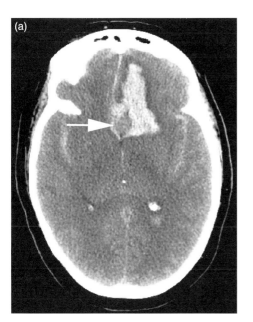 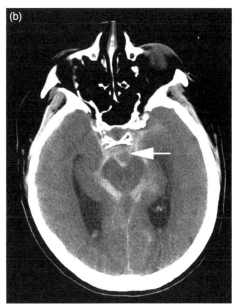

Fig. 7.2. (a) Axial image demonstrating extensive hyperdense blood in the left frontal lobe, interhemispheric fissure, Sylvian fissures bilaterally and occipital horn, secondary to rupture of an anterior communication artery aneurysm (arrow). (b) Axial image demonstrating extensive hyperdense blood within the interpeduncular and ambient cisterns secondary to rupture of a basilar artery tip aneurysm (arrow).

- Uses a combination of multiplanar reformat, maximal intensity projection (Fig 7.3b), and volume and surface rendering from the source images. This allows identification and depiction of aneurysm anatomy including: aneurysm location, size, neck, orientation, and relationship to parent vessel, adjacent vessels and other structures. The anatomy will determine patient management with endovascular coiling or surgical clipping.
- Best performed by experienced radiologists using protocols agreed with a neurosurgical centre.

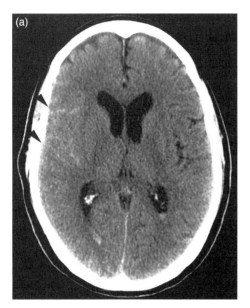 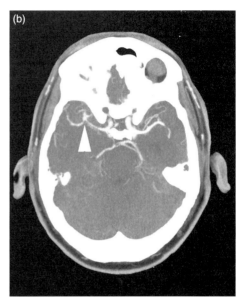

Fig. 7.3. (a) Axial image demonstrating subtle hyperdense subarachnoid blood within the right convexity sulci (black arrowheads). There is layering of blood in the occipital horns of the lateral ventricles. (b) Maximum-intensity projection image from a CT angiogram showing small right MCA aneurysm (arrowhead).

Chapter

8

Cerebral venous sinus thrombosis

Characteristics

- A rare cause of stroke, more common in younger age groups, with a female preponderance.
- Risk factors:

Septic causes (especially in children)
  - Intracranial infections: meningitis, encephalitis, brain abscess, empyema
  - Locoregional infection: mastoiditis.

Aseptic causes
  - Hypercoagulable states: polycythaemia rubra vera, idiopathic thrombocytosis.
  - Hormonal: pregnancy, oral contraceptive pill.

Trauma
  - Head injury
  - Iatrogenic procedures: lumbar puncture, neurosurgical intervention.

Low flow state
  - Dehydration. (especially in children)

Clinical features

- Sudden-onset severe headache (75%) – may mimic SAH.
- Focal neurological deficit (50%).
- Seizures, nausea and vomiting frequently occur.
- Often non-specific presentation. Cerebral venous sinus thrombosis should be considered in young patients with headache or stroke-like symptoms without any vascular risk factors.

Radiological features

CT

- CT scan without contrast should be performed initially to rule out haemorrhagic-related causes. This can then be followed by a contrast-enhanced scan.

Features

- CT may be normal.

Non-contrast CT

- Thrombus appears hyperdense for the first 7–14 days, after which time it is isodense.
- Thrombus within a cerebral vein: linear hyperdense material within a vessel representing thrombosed blood (Fig. 8.1).

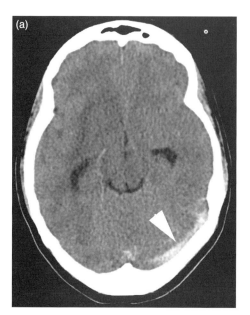 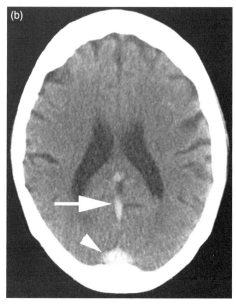

Fig. 8.1. Axial images showing high-density acute thrombus within the (a) left transverse sinus (arrowhead); (b) straight sinus (arrow), and torcula (arrowhead).

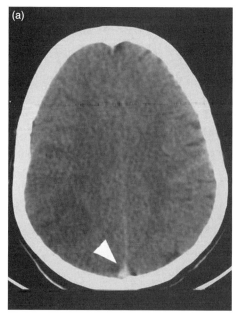 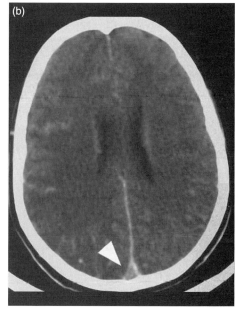

Fig. 8.2. Axial images: (a) pre-contrast image showing hyperdense acute thrombus within the posterior sagittal sinus – the *delta sign* (arrowhead); (b) post-contrast image demonstrating contrast outlining the thrombus – the *empty delta sign* (arrowhead).

- Superior sagittal sinus thrombosis: classically hyperdense triangle within the sinus known as the *delta sign* (Fig. 8.2a).
- Low-attenuation areas of cerebral infarction not conforming to an arterial territory.
- Signs of infection such as sinuitis/mastoiditis, which can be complicated by venous sinus thrombosis.

Contrast CT

- Thrombus will appear as a filling defect surrounded by enhancing dura.
- Superior sagittal sinus thrombosis – look for the *empty delta sign* (seen in 70% of cases) (Fig. 8.2b).

MRI

Features

- Absence of normal flow void on T1- and T2-weighted images (Fig. 8.3a). Signal characteristics are dependent on the age of the thrombus.
- Acute thrombus (up to 5 days): isointense on T1, hypointense on T2.
- Subacute thrombus (5–15 days): hyperintense on T1 and T2.
- Thrombus and venous infarction appear hyperintense on FLAIR.
- Haemorrhagic foci: best seen on gradient echo imaging due to susceptibility-induced signal loss from deoxyhaemoglobin.
- Post-contrast T1: peripheral enhancement surrounding the thrombus.
- MR venography: absence of normal flow voids (Fig. 8.3b, c).

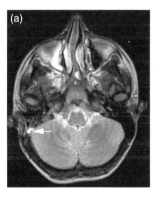

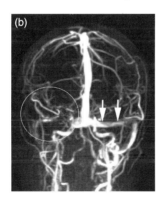

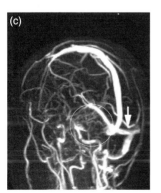

Fig. 8.3. (a) Axial T2W MR brain image demonstrating high signal within the right transverse sinus (arrow) consistent with absent flow void secondary to thrombosis; (b) and (c) phase-contrast MR venography demonstrating absence of signal within the right transverse sinus due to thrombosis (circle) vs. normal flow in the left transverse sinus (arrows).

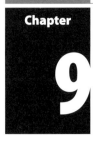

Chapter

9 Traumatic parenchymal brain injury

Characteristics

- Traumatic injury resulting in neuronal and vascular injury; can occur in the presence of other types of intracranial haemorrhage.
- Incidence is difficult to assess, as patients with mild injury do not present, while those with severe injury often die at the scene of the incident and are therefore under-reported.
- Usually results from linear acceleration/deceleration forces or penetrating injuries.
- Can be subcategorized into: primary injury, including contusion and diffuse axonal injury, and secondary injury, including diffuse cerebral oedema and brain herniation.

Clinical features

- Patients often present with a history of head trauma or external signs of injury.
- Usually associated with a brief loss of consciousness.
- Confusion and altered GCS may be prolonged.
- Headache with vomiting in the conscious patient.
- Focal neurological deficit may occur if contusions arise near the sensorimotor cortex.
- Most patients make an uneventful recovery, but a few develop raised intracranial pressure, post-traumatic seizures and persisting focal neurological deficits.

Radiological features

CT

- CT scan without contrast, as high-density contrast may obscure visualization of blood.

Features
Contusion

- Solitary or multiple foci of high-density haematomas in the cortical or subcortical region, representing primary parenchymal and vascular injuries (Fig. 9.1).
- Most commonly located in the anterior, lateral and inferior surfaces of the frontal and temporal lobes; thought to be related to the relative irregularity of the skull base at these sites.

- Parenchymal injury adjacent to site of external trauma is termed *coup injury*. A *contracoup injury* results from impact of the moving brain against the inner skull table, opposite to the site of direct injury. Paradoxically, this is often more severe than the coup injury.

- The resulting cell damage leads to cytotoxic brain oedema, resulting in regional ischaemia, appearing as hypodense areas of brain parenchyma in association with the high-density contusion.

Diffuse axonal injury

- Small and multiple lesions of high attenuation secondary to the widespread disruption of axons during acceleration/deceleration injury.

- Typically located in the corpus callosal complex, parasagittal grey–white matter junction, deep periventricular white matter (especially in the frontal areas), basal ganglia, internal capsule, hippocampal and para-hippocampal regions, brainstem and cerebellum (Fig. 9.2).

- Focal haematomas and diffuse axonal injury are more accurately assessed with MR imaging than with CT. A gradient recall echo sequence is recommended because of its ability to detect susceptibility artefacts from haemosiderin secondary to haemorrhage. However, this is infrequently used in the acute setting due to the length of examination and safety risks incurred during patient transfer.

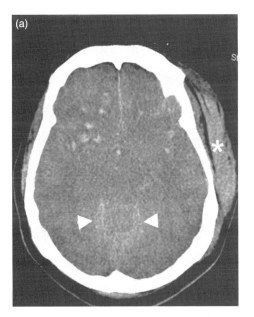 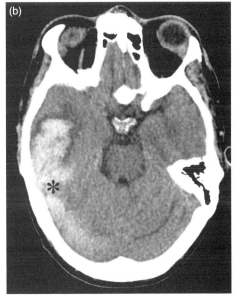

Fig. 9.1. Axial images demonstrating (a) multifocal contusions within both frontal lobes, with additional acute subarachnoid haemorrhage along the basal cisterns and tentorium (arrowheads), marked frontoparietal soft-tissue swelling (asterisk); (b) large right temporal contusion.

Diffuse cerebral oedema

- Results from either hyperaemia or interstitial oedema. Leads to effacement of sulci, loss of the suprasellar and quadrigeminal cisterns, and compression of the ventricles.
- Generalized homogeneous low-attenuation parenchyma represents a diffuse loss of grey–white matter differentiation secondary to oedema. The cerebellum may appear hyperdense in comparison: *white cerebellum sign* (Fig. 9.3a).

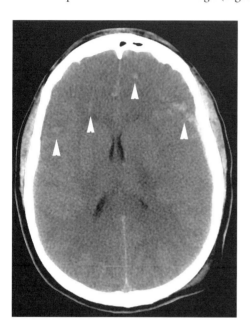

Fig. 9.2. Axial image showing multiple subtle areas of high attenuation in the frontal lobes bilaterally (arrowheads) at grey–white matter junctions and deep white matter, in keeping with diffuse axonal injury.

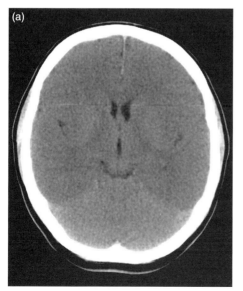
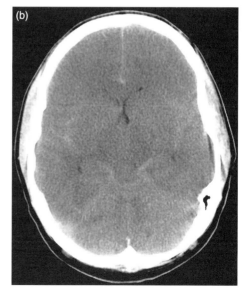

Fig. 9.3. Axial images showing diffuse low attenuation cerebral parenchyma causing (a) relative hyperdensity of the cerebellum – *white cerebellum sign*; (b) relative hyperdensity of the blood vessels and meninges and effacement of the basal cisterns – *pseudo-subarachnoid haemorrhage appearance*.

- The diffuse low density of the cerebrum can produce a *pseudo-subarachnoid haemorrhage appearance*, as the dura and vessels appear relatively hyperdense against the brain parenchyma (Fig. 9.3b).

Brain herniation

- *Subfalcine herniation* – displacement of the cingulate gyrus across the midline under the falx. The anterior cerebral artery is displaced, resulting in secondary ischaemia and infarction (Fig. 9.4).

- *Transtentorial herniation* – downward displacement of temporal lobes and brainstem leading to effacement of the basal cisterns, dilatation of the contralateral ventricular system due to obstruction to CSF flow, and midline shift of the brain parenchyma (Fig. 9.5).

- *Tonsillar herniation* – cerebellar tonsils are displaced inferiorly through the foramen magnum. Look for loss of the low-density CSF fluid around the brainstem at this level (Fig. 9.6).

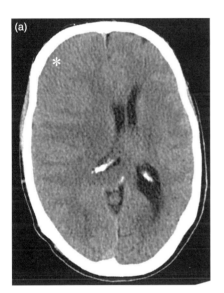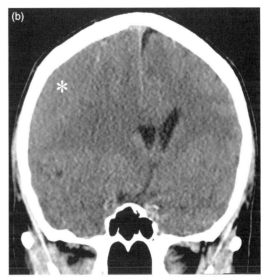

Fig. 9.4. (a) Axial and (b) coronal images showing subfalcine herniation secondary to mass effect from subacute subdural haematoma (asterix).

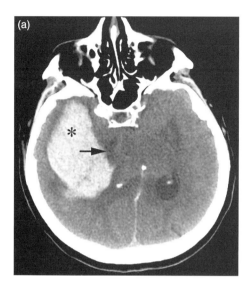
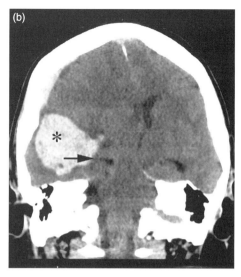

Fig. 9.5. (a) Axial and (b) coronal images showing transtentorial herniation with effacement of the basal cisterns secondary to a right intraparenchymal haematoma (asterix). Black arrow indicates the medially displaced temporal horn of the right lateral ventricle. There is also evidence of subfalcine herniation and a right-sided subdural haematoma.

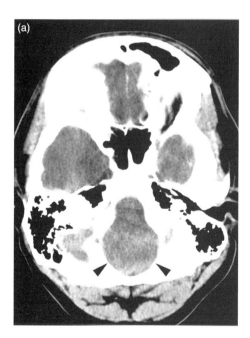

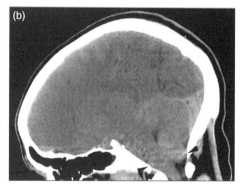

Fig. 9.6. (a) Axial and (b) sagittal images showing tonsillar herniation with complete effacement of the CSF space at the level of the foramen magnum (arrowheads).

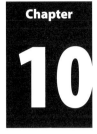

Chapter

10 Hydrocephalus

Characteristics

Hydrocephalus is an accumulation of CSF in the brain, which results from an imbalance between CSF production and absorption.

- Communicating hydrocephalus

  Reduced CSF absorption
  - Obstruction at the level of pacchionian granulations
  - SAH, meningitis, venous thrombosis

  Increased CSF production
  - Choroid plexus tumours

  Normal pressure hydrocephalus
  - Clinical triad: gait disturbance, dementia and urinary incontinence.
  - No evidence of raised intracranial pressure
- Non-communicating hydrocephalus
  - Obstruction of the ventricles, foraminae or aqueduct, causing dilatation proximal to the obstruction with normal calibre distal to the obstruction.

Causes

- *Foramen of Monro*
  - Colloid cyst of the third ventricle, oligodendroglioma, ependymoma, suprasellar tumours, giant cell astrocytoma (tuberous sclerosis).
- *Aqueduct of Sylvius*
  - Congenital aqueduct stenosis, intraventricular haemorrhage, ventriculitis.
- *Fourth ventricle/foraminae of Luschka and Magendie*
  - Congenital: Dandy–Walker malformation, intraventricular haemorrhage, posterior fossa tumours: ependymoma, medulloblastoma, haemangioblastoma.

Clinical features

- Neonate/infant

  o Enlarged cranium, bulging fontanelles, widely separated cranial sutures, vomiting, drowsiness, irritability, eyes turned downwards due to paralysis of upward gaze.

- Older children and adults

  o Headaches, nausea, vomiting, papilloedema, diplopia, problems with balance and coordination, gait disturbance, urinary incontinence

Radiological features

CT

Features
Communicating hydrocephalus

- Symmetrical enlargement of the ventricles.
- Mass effect causing effacement of sulci.
- Periventricular interstitial oedema.

Non-communicating hydrocephalus

- Disproportionate dilatation of the ventricles proximal to the obstruction.
- Abnormality causing the obstruction (Fig. 10.1).

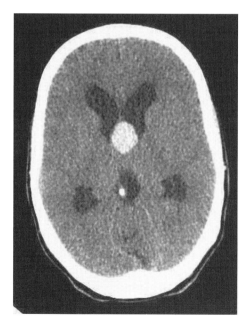

Fig. 10.1. Axial image showing obstructive hydrocephalus, secondary to a hyperdense colloid cyst at the level of the foramen of Monro. There is resultant mass effect with dilatation of both frontal horns and trigones of the lateral ventricles, and generalized effacement of the cerebral sulci.

- Grossly dilated temporal horns of the lateral ventricles.
- Mass effect causing effacement of the sulci.
- Periventricular low-attenuation interstitial oedema from venous congestion (Fig. 10.2).

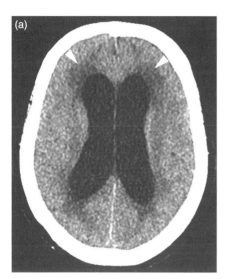 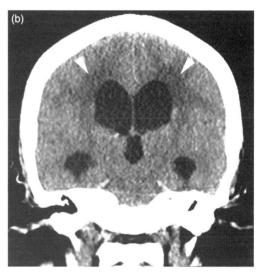

Fig. 10.2. (a) Axial and (b) coronal images showing symmetrical dilatation of the lateral ventricles, and ballooning of the third ventricle. There is periventricular low-attenuation interstitial oedema (arrowheads). Note also generalized effacement of the extra-axial spaces.

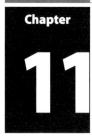

Chapter

Hypoxic-ischaemic injury (HII)

Characteristics

- Results from all causes leading to diminished cerebral blood flow (ischaemia) and reduced blood oxygenation (hypoxaemia).
- Affects all age groups, from premature infants to adults. The pattern of damage is determined by the degree of brain maturity, metabolic activity in the area of affected brain, severity and duration of the hypoxic-ischaemic insult.
- Asphyxia is the most common cause in infants, with cardiac arrest being the leading cause in adults.
- A devastating condition, which can result in severe long-term neurological disability and death.
- Imaging helps to secure an early diagnosis, enabling intervention in the acute stage. Information on severity and extent of injury in the subacute setting helps to predict long-term outcome.

Clinical features

Term and preterm neonates

- Related to antepartum (maternal hypotension, multiple gestations and prenatal infection) or intrapartum risk factors (forceps delivery, breech extraction or placental abruption).
- Premature neonates are more vulnerable to perinatal insults, leading to hypoperfusion.
- Imaging plays an important role in distinguishing between neurological immaturity and IIII, as clinical signs can be confusing.

Children and adults

- HII in adults often results from cardiac arrest or cerebrovascular disease.
- Drowning and asphyxiation are the more common causes in older children.

Post-anoxic leucoencephalopathy

- A specific but uncommon cause of delayed white-matter injury occurring weeks after the hypoxic-ischaemic event, most commonly associated with carbon monoxide poisoning.
- Can also manifest as progressive deterioration in neurology.

- Delirium, personality change, intellectual impairment, movement disorders or seizures may be present.

Radiological features

Cranial ultrasound

Features

- Useful in infants below 4 months of age, where the anterior fontanelle offers a window for imaging.
- Increased cerebral echogenicity is seen in the affected area, with varying patterns depending on the age and severity of the injury. Periventricular leucomalacia and germinal matrix haemorrhage are specific findings related to mild asphyxia in premature infants.
- Delayed findings include cerebral atrophy, with prominence of the ventricles and extraaxial CSF-containing spaces.

CT

Features

- Early CT may appear 'normal', with subtle low-density change in the deep grey matter.
- Subsequent changes include cortical hypoattenuation, loss of normal grey–white matter differentiation, and diffuse cerebral oedema, with cisternal and sulcal effacement.
- The *reversal sign* may be seen within the first 24 hours, with higher attenuation of the white matter compared with the cortical grey matter.
- The *white cerebellum sign*, caused by diffuse oedema, may be observed, resulting in hypoattenuation of the cerebral hemispheres with sparing of the cerebellum and brainstem (Fig. 11.1).

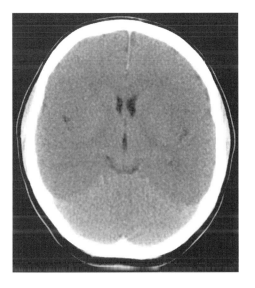

Fig. 11.1. Axial CT brain image demonstrating complete loss of cerebral grey–white matter differentiation, with relative increase in attenuation of the cerebellum, due to diffuse oedema of the cerebral hemispheres – *white cerebellum sign*.

MRI

Features

- Conventional T1- and T2-weighted images may initially appear normal, with subsequent variable signal change over the first few weeks following the injury (Fig. 11.2a).

- Diffusion-weighted imaging (DWI) is the most sensitive sequence in HII in the first 24 hours (Fig. 11.2b, c), demonstrating high signal intensity in vulnerable areas, which varies depending on the severity of the asphyxia. This often underestimates the extent of the injury and follow-up delayed imaging is necessary.

- These techniques, while useful, are best left in the hands of an experienced radiologist. Non-contrast CT becomes the initial imaging study of choice in postnatal infants, children and adults.

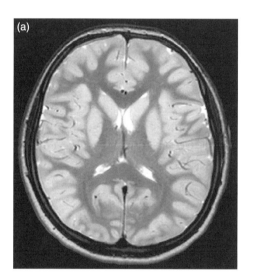

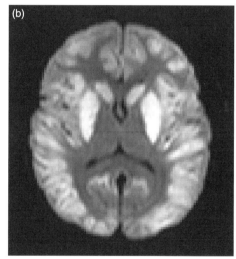

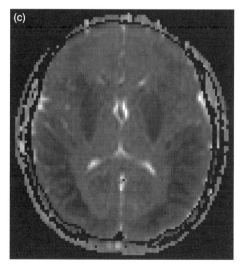

Fig. 11.2. MRI of the brain: (a) T2W imaging demonstrating extensive hyperintensity and swelling of the cortical surfaces of both hemispheres and basal ganglia; (b) DWI demonstrating high signal in these areas, with corresponding low signal on the (c) ADC map. The appearances are consistent with cortical and basal ganglia infarction secondary to severe ischaemia.

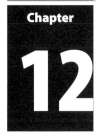

Meningitis

Characteristics

- Inflammation of the meninges, which can be further divided anatomically into:
  - *Pachymeningitis* – inflammation of the dura
  - *Leptomeningitis* – inflammation of the arachnoid membrane and subarachnoid space
  - *Meningoencephalitis* – inflammation extending to involve the parenchyma.
- Widespread use of the haemophilus influenzae B, pneumocococcal and meningococcal C vaccines have reduced the incidence of meningitis in children.
- The median age of patients has risen to 25 years and it has become a disease of young adults.
- Concurrent illness such as pneumonia or other sites of sepsis (e.g. sinusitis, mastoiditis, otitis media) may extend directly to involve the meninges.

Clinical features

- Presentation with fever, stiff neck, photophobia, headache and cerebral dysfunction, although common, is not specific for meningitis.
- Kernig's and Brudzinski's signs indicate the presence of meningeal irritation.
- Seizures, cranial nerve palsies and signs of raised intracranial pressure, such as papilloedema and Cushing reflex, may also be present.
- Detection at the extremes of age is difficult. Children may present with poor feeding, irritability, lethargy and vomiting. The elderly may only have a low-grade fever and delirium.
- CSF sampling for Gram stain, white cell count, glucose and protein will confirm the diagnosis. CT of the head is required prior to lumbar puncture in the presence of depressed consciousness or focal neurological deficit.

Radiological features

CT

- CT scan without contrast should be performed in the first instance to rule out a haemorrhagic cause of the symptoms.

Features
Non-contrast CT

- Often normal in the early phase.

- Subtle meningeal thickening with increased density may be present.

- Features of secondary complications such as abscess, cerebral oedema, raised intracranial pressure, hydrocephalus and venous sinus thrombosis may be present.

- Reduction in size of the basal and suprasellar cisterns with sulcal effacement is suggestive of cerebral oedema and raised intracranial pressure.

- A primary infective source may be identified in the study, e.g. sinusitis and mastoiditis. Check on bone windows for bone destruction.

Contrast-enhanced CT

- Enhancement of the meningeal surfaces is non-specific, and is often an inconsistent finding in patients with meningitis. Best seen over the cerebral convexities and in the interhemispheric and Sylvian fissures (Fig. 12.1).

- Intense contrast enhancement of the thickened meninges, noted on the non-contrast CT, is suggestive of granulomatous meningitis, as seen in tuberculosis (TB) or sarcoidosis.

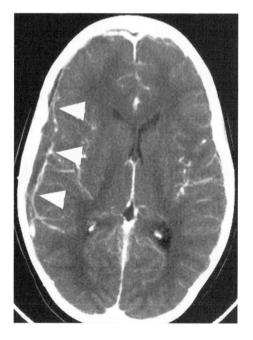

Fig. 12.1. Axial image demonstrating meningeal enhancement (arrowheads) in a patient with pneumococcal meningitis, with a concurrent subdural empyema.

Chapter

13

Encephalitis

Characteristics

- Inflammation of the brain parenchyma.
- Most commonly due to a viral infection resulting in parenchymal damage of varying severity.
- If untreated, has a mortality of 50–75%, with long-term motor and mental disabilities in most – if not all – of the survivors.
- *Herpes simplex* virus is the most common sporadic cause, with varicella-zoster virus and cytomegalovirus being common in immunocompromised hosts.
- Brain infection can arise from haematological spread, or by direct neuronal transmission via the trigeminal or olfactory nerve. This can occur as a result of reactivation of a latent infection.

Clinical features

- Signs and symptoms may mimic those of meningitis and are often indistinguishable from it.
- Presentation may include behavioural and personality changes, decreased level of consciousness, and acute confusion.
- Viral prodrome including fever, headache, nausea and vomiting, lethargy and myalgias may also be reported.
- There may be hemiparesis, ataxia, cranial nerve defects and meningism. A careful search for signs of viral infection can help to support the diagnosis.
- Confirmation of the diagnosis is performed by polymerase chain reaction (PCR) testing of CSF or identification of the virus from a brain biopsy.

Radiological features

CT

Features

- May appear normal in the early phase.
- *Herpes simplex* encephalitis has a predilection for the inferior frontal and inferio-medial temporal lobes. Characteristically, the parenchyma appears hypodense and may be missed if bilateral (Fig. 13.1).

- Signs of cerebral oedema may develop in severe cases due to inflammation.
- Contrast administration may demonstrate a gyral pattern of enhancement in the temporal and parietal lobes.

MRI

Features

- A more sensitive investigation, with characteristic changes demonstrated at an earlier stage.
- Ill-defined reduced T1 and increased T2 signal involving the frontal and temporal lobes, as outlined above (Fig. 13.2).
- Gyral enhancement may also be seen on contrast-enhanced images.

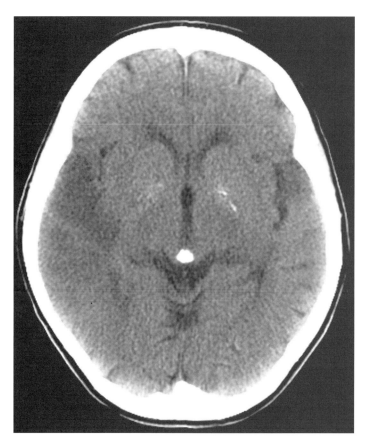

Fig. 13.1. Axial CT image demonstrating bilateral low attenuation in the temporal lobes secondary to *Herpes simplex* encephalitis.

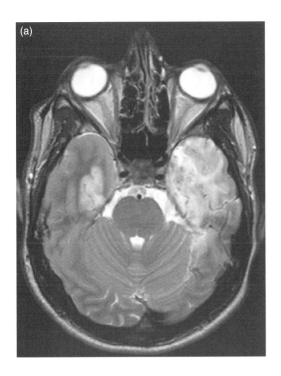

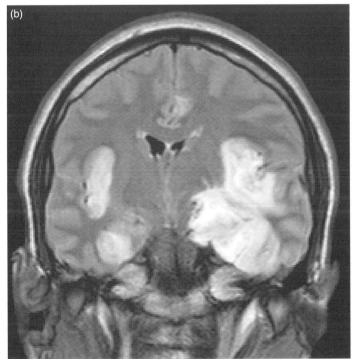

Fig. 13.2. (a) Axial T2W MRI of the brain demonstrating high signal within the anterior temporal lobes bilaterally. (b) Coronal FLAIR MRI of the brain demonstrating high signal within the medial temporal lobes and extending into the insula cortex bilaterally. The appearance is consistent with *Herpes simplex* encephalitis.

Chapter

14

Cerebral abscess

Characteristics

- Localized purulent bacterial infection developing in an area of cerebritis.

Causes

- Septic emboli transmitted haematogenously (e.g. secondary to endocarditis).
- Transdural spread from adjacent sinus infection.
- Penetrating trauma or surgery.

Predisposing factors

- Diabetes mellitus, steroids/immunosuppressive therapy, immune deficiency.

Causative organisms

- Anaerobic Streptococcus (most common), Staphylococcus, Bacteroides.
- Multiple organisms in 20% of cases.
- Mycobacterium and/or Salmonella – more common in developing countries.
- Toxoplasmosis in immunocompromised patients.

Clinical features

- Headache, vomiting, seizures, altered mental state and spiking pyrexia.
- Cranial nerve palsies or localized peripheral neurological deficits.
- Signs of raised intracranial pressure.
- Identifiable source of sepsis or pyrexia of unknown origin.
- Diagnosis and treatment is difficult in those who are immunosuppressed.
- Significant long-term morbidity.

Radiological features

CT

- The initial CT scan should be performed without contrast to rule out a haemorrhagic cause of symptoms. Subsequent scan with contrast can then be performed.

Features

- Typically at the corticomedullary junction in the frontal and temporal lobes.

Non-contrast CT

- Low-attenuation lesion with associated mass effect.
- Gas within the lesion from gas-forming organisms.

Contrast-enhanced CT

- Thin-walled ring enhancement (2–7 mm) with a smooth convex surface (Fig. 14.1) (compared with a thick, irregular wall in a cerebral neoplasm).
- Central low-attenuation necrosis, which does not fill with contrast.
- Surrounding low-attenuation oedema causing mass effect.
- Lesions may be multi-loculated, and adjacent daughter abscesses may develop.
- Extension into the ventricles can result in ventriculitis. This is confirmed by an increase in attenuation of CSF fluid within the ventricles, with associated ependymal enhancement (Fig. 14.2).

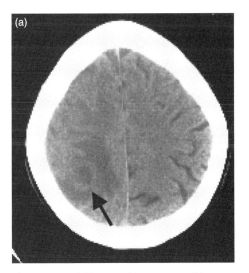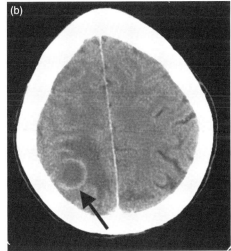

Fig. 14.1. Axial CT images: (a) pre-contrast (b) post-contrast, showing right superior parietal ring enhancing lesion (black arrows) with surrounding vasogenic oedema.

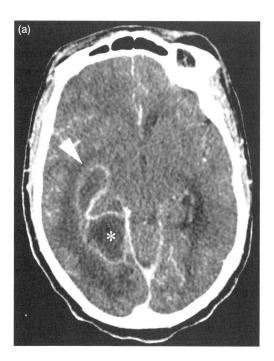

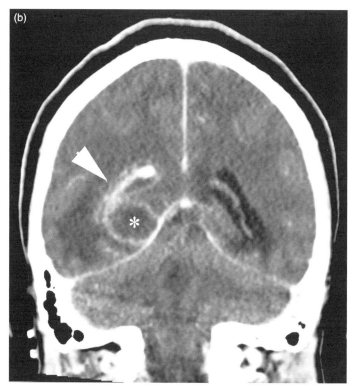

Fig. 14.2. Post-contrast (a) axial and (b) coronal CT images showing a right intracerebral abscess (asterix) with rim enhancement; note the ependymal enhancement in the adjacent ventricle in keeping with ventriculitis (arrowhead).

MRI

Features

- Abscess rim is typically hypointense on T2-weighted images (Fig. 14.3a).
- Avid rim enhancement post contrast (Fig. 14.3b).
- Restricted diffusion on DWI (high signal on DWI, low signal on ADC) (Fig. 14.3c, d).

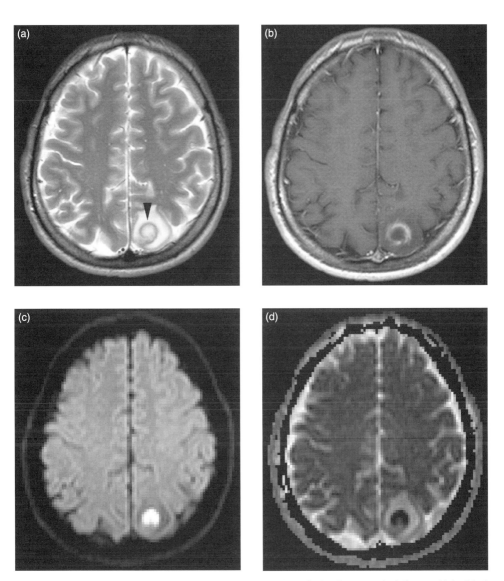

Fig. 14.3. MRI of the brain: (a) T2W imaging demonstrating thick rim fluid collection in the left parietal lobe (black arrowhead) with surrounding vasogenic oedema; (b) T1W imaging post contrast, showing avid rim enhancement; (c) DWI and (d) ADC demonstrating high and low signal, respectively, confirming restricted diffusion within the collection in keeping with abscess.

Arteriovenous malformation

15

Characteristics

- Congenital abnormality secondary to failure of embryonic vascular plexus differentiation.

- Cerebral vascular lesions allow low-pressure direct shunting of blood from the arterial to the venous system, without an intervening capillary bed, resulting in enlarged feeding vessels and draining veins.

- Accounts for 11% of cerebrovascular malformations and may be part of a congenital syndrome, e.g. Sturge–Weber, neurofibromatosis or von Hippel–Lindau syndrome.

- Venous malformations are less common, e.g. medullary venous and cavernous malformations. Arteriovenous fistulae are usually post-traumatic.

Clinical features

- Often asymptomatic and clinically silent until the presenting event, although 10% are diagnosed incidentally.

- Minor cognitive impairment in up to two-thirds of patients, although largely subclinical and often do not come to medical attention.

- Headaches may be reported in up to half of all patients and may take the form of migraines.

- May present with seizures (non-focal in 40%), acute intracranial haemorrhage, or progressive neurological deficit. Rarely, focal neurological deficit may indicate the site of an AVM.

Radiological features

CT

- Non-contrast CT should be used initially, as high-density contrast may mask underlying haemorrhage.

Location

- Supratentorial (90%): parietal > frontal > temporal > occipital lobe.
- Infratentorial (10%).

Vascular supply

- Pial branches of the internal carotid artery (ICA) in 75% of supratentorial lesions and in 50% of posterior fossa lesions.
- Dural branches of the external carotid artery (ECA) in 25% of infratentorial lesions.

Features

Unenhanced CT

- Cerebral or extra-axial haemorrhage. Secondary signs of AVM, including dilated dural sinuses and draining cerebral veins may be seen, although these are better demonstrated post contrast.
- 10% of AVM are not visualized on unenhanced CT.
- Lesions can appear as an isoattenuating to hyperattenuating mass:
  - *Mixed-density lesion* (60%), composed of large dense vessels, haemorrhage and calcification (Fig. 15.1)
  - *Isodense lesion* (15%), which may only be recognizable by associated mass effect
  - *Low-density lesion* (15%), due to encephalomalacia, atrophy or gliosis secondary to associated local cerebral ischaemia.

Contrast-enhanced CT

- AVMs may enhance, with dense serpiginous enhancement representing tortuous dilated vessels in 80% of cases (Fig. 15.2).
- Adjacent low attenuation may be present due to oedema, mass effect or ischaemic changes.

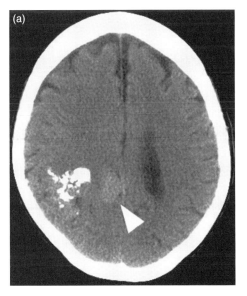 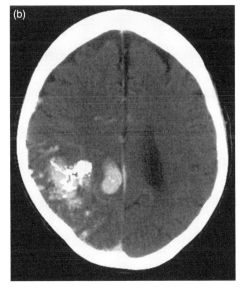

Fig. 15.1. Axial CT images: (a) pre-contrast and (b) post-contrast showing a mixed-density lesion composed of coarse calcification and faintly hyperdense vessels (arrowhead). There is marked enhancement within the tortuous vessels post contrast.

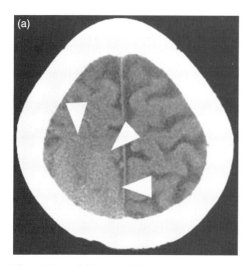 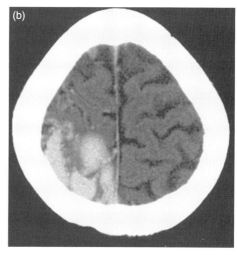

Fig. 15.2. Axial CT images: (a) pre-contrast and (b) post-contrast showing large faintly hyperdense cortical vessels seen at the right vertex (arrowheads) with marked enhancement post contrast.

CT angiography

Features

- Demonstrates the presence of a nidus and venous shunting to confirm diagnosis.
- Despite advances in spatial and temporal resolution, delineation of feeding arteries and draining veins is technically difficult. Cerebral angiography is therefore required for haemodynamic assessment and treatment planning.

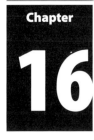

Chapter

16

Solitary lesions

Characteristics

- Solitary space-occupying lesions are frequently tumours.
- One-third are metastases from breast, lung or melanoma primaries.
- Most commonly found in the cerebral hemisphere at the grey–white matter junction.
- Primary tumours (e.g. astrocytoma, glioblastoma multiforme, oligodendrogliomas, ependymomas) have <50% 5-year survival. Two-thirds are supratentorial in adults, while two-thirds are infratentorial in children.
- Other solitary lesions included in the differential diagnosis are cerebral abscesses, aneurysms, tuberculomas, granulomas and cysts.

Clinical features

- Seizures are a common first presentation in adults.
- Focal neurology may evolve with increasing size of the lesion or associated mass effect.
- Tumours usually run an indolent course and rarely cause a sudden increase in intracranial pressure.
- Solitary mass lesions can cause local effects, e.g. proptosis or epistaxis.
- Clinical presentation may help localize the site of the lesion:
  - *Frontal lobe* – hemiparesis, seizures, personality change, grasp reflex (unilateral is significant), expressive dysphasia (Broca's area) and anosmia.
  - *Temporal lobe* – complex partial seizures, hallucinations, feelings of déjà vu, taste, smell, dysphasia (Wernicke's area), visual field defects, fugue, functional psychosis.
  - *Parietal lobe* – hemisensory loss, decreased stereognosis, sensory inattention, dysphasia and Gerstmann's syndrome (finger agnosia, left/right disorientation, dysgraphia, acalculia).
  - *Occipital lobe* – contralateral visual field defects.
  - *Cerebellum* – past-pointing, intention tremor, nystagmus, dysdiadochokinesis and truncal ataxia (worse if eyes open).
  - *Cerebellopontine angle* – nystagmus, reduced corneal reflex, fifth and seventh cranial nerve palsies, ipsilateral cerebellar signs and ipsilateral deafness.

    ○ *Mid-brain* – unequal pupils, confabulation, somnolence and an inability to direct the eyes up or down.

Radiological features

CT

Features

- The age of the patient and lesion location will aid the differential diagnosis, although often not vital in the emergency setting.
- Cerebral masses encompass a spectrum of appearances (Table 16.1):
  - *Density*: lesions may be hypo-, iso- or hyperdense.
  - *Calcification*: if present may indicate a less aggressive pathology
  - *Contrast enhancement*: often helpful in lesion characterisation. In cases of rim enhancement, abscess should be excluded (Fig. 16.1).
- Important to identify complications such as haemorrhage, cerebral oedema, hydrocephalus and cerebellar tonsillar herniation.

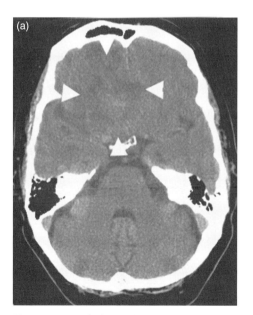 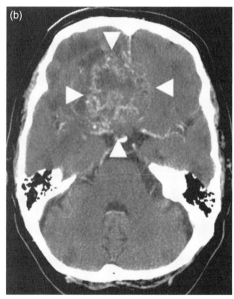

Fig. 16.1. Frontal glioma (a) pre-contrast and (b) post-contrast axial images showing ill defined areas of low attenuation within the right frontal lobe (arrowheads). There is significant enhancement post contrast, with central low attenuation in keeping with necrosis. There is associated peripheral low-density oedema.

Table 16.1 CT imaging features of some commonly seen lesions.

Lesion	Location	Density	Calcification	Contrast enhancement
Haematoma <1 week	Variable	↑	–	–
Haematoma 1–2 weeks	Variable	↔	–	–
Haematoma >2 weeks	Variable	↓	Occasional	–
Colloid cysts	Foramen of Monro	↑ (80%)/ ↔ (20%)	–	Peripheral
Arachnoid cyst	Anterior temporal lobe (50%)	↓	–	–
Giant aneurysm	Cavernous/supraclinoid ICA, basilar	↑	Curvilinear	Target sign
Pyogenic abscess	Variable	↓	–	Ring enhancement
Meningioma (Fig. 16.2)	Supratentorial (90%), extra-axial	↑ (70%)	Circular or radial	Intense uniform
Ependymoma (NF)	Floor of 4th ventricle	↔/ mildly ↑	Occasionally punctate	Solid component only
Primary lymphoma (HIV)	Periventricular, crosses the midline	↑	–	Homogeneous
Metastases	Corticomedullary junction, multiple	↓ (unless haemorrhagic)		Solid/ring-like
Glioblastoma multiforme (Fig. 16.3)	Frontal/temporal lobe, callosal	↓/↔/↑ (haemorrhage)	Rarely	Homo/ heterogeneous, ring pattern
Medulloblastoma	Cerebellum; vermis and roof of 4th ventricle	↑ (70%)	Rarely (13%)	Intense homogeneous
Vestibular schwannoma (NF2)	Cerebellopontine angle	↔/↓	–	Uniform dense/ ring-like
Haemangioblastoma (VHL)	Paravermian cerebellar hemisphere (85%)	↓ (Cystic)	–	Peripheral mural/ solid enhancing
Epidermoid	Cerebellopontine angle (40%)	↓	25%	Peripheral
Dermoid	Posterior fossa (vermis)/ 4th ventricle	↓ (Fat content)	Mural/central	–
Craniopharyngioma	Multilobular suprasellar (50%)	↔ (54–75%)	Marginal	Peripheral if cystic/ enhances if solid

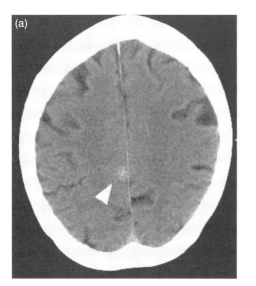
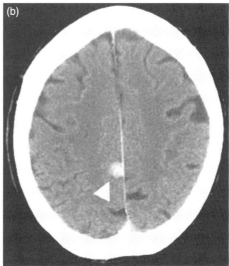

Fig. 16.2. Right parafalcine meningioma: (a) pre-contrast and (b) post-contrast axial images showing a faintly hyperdense extra-axial lesion prior to contrast, which enhances avidly post contrast (arrowhead).

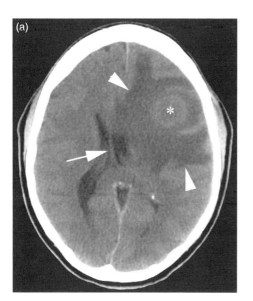
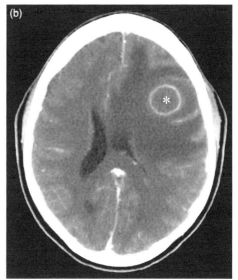

Fig. 16.3. Left glioblastoma multiforme: axial images (a) pre-contrast and (b) post-contrast showing a left frontal lesion (asterix) with extensive surrounding oedema (arrowheads). There is significant mass effect with midline shift to the right (arrow) and avid rim enhancement post contrast.

Chapter

17

Multiple lesions

Characteristics

- The differential diagnosis of multiple lesions include:
  - ○ *Neoplastic:* Metastases (Figs. 17.1 and 17.2 a, b, c) are the most common intracerebral neoplastic lesion (lung, breast, melanoma, renal, colon primaries). Found in up to 24% of all patients who die from cancer. Represents 20–30% of all brain tumours in adults.
  - ○ *Infective:* Cerebral abscesses (Fig. 17.3a, b), granulomata (Fig. 17.2d).
  - ○ *Vascular:* Multiple lesions of varying age are seen in multi-infarct dementia.
  - ○ *Inflammatory:* Demyelinating plaques can be seen as multiple low-density lesions on CT, predominantly in the periventricular deep white matter.
  - ○ *Traumatic:* Contusions are frequently multiple after head trauma.

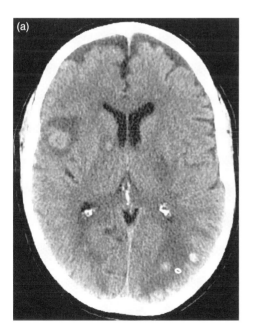

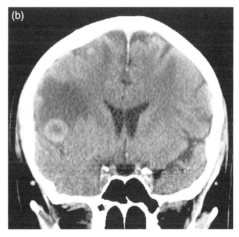

Fig. 17.1. (a) Axial and (b) coronal unenhanced CT images demonstrating multiple hyperdense lesions with marked surrounding vasogenic oedema. Appearances are in keeping with metastases from melanoma.

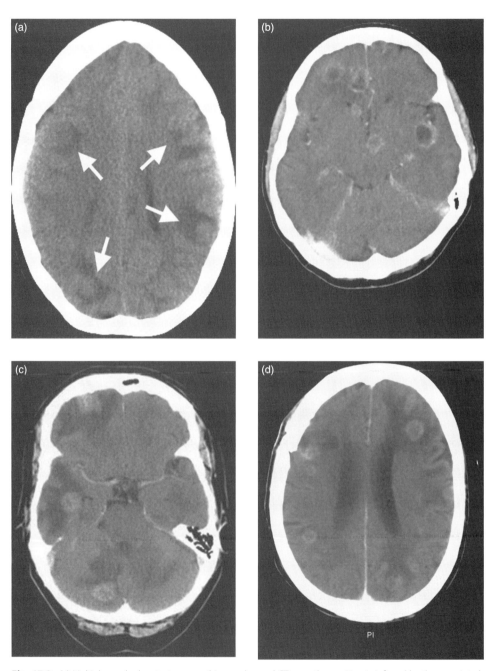

Fig. 17.2. (a) Multiple cerebral metastases: on this unenhanced CT scan, the position is inferred by the associated oedema (arrows). (b) Multiple necrotic metastases with thick irregular rim enhancement. (c) Multiple solid enhancing metastases with surrounding vasogenic oedema. (d) Multiple tuberculomas showing thick irregular rim enhancement.

Clinical and radiological features

- Dependent on the underlying pathology. Please refer to Chapter 16 (Solitary lesions).

Radiological features

CT

Features

- Damage to the blood–brain barrier results in varying degrees of lesion enhancement. The pattern of enhancement may narrow the differential diagnosis.

- Melanoma metastases classically appear hyperdense prior to contrast enhancement (Fig. 17.1).

- Calcification in malignant tumours is uncommon. If present, this suggests metasteses from mucinous tumours of the gastrointestinal (GI) tract or breast, or cartilage/bone-forming sarcomas. Haemorrhage into metastases occurs infrequently, and when present suggests hypervascular tumours such as melanoma or renal cell carcinoma.

- Calcification following granulomatous infection is not uncommon.

- Cerebral contusions may be rather inconspicuous on initial CT, usually becoming more apparent on interval CT at about 2 weeks.

- MRI is much more sensitive in detecting contusions and should be considered if not contraindicated.

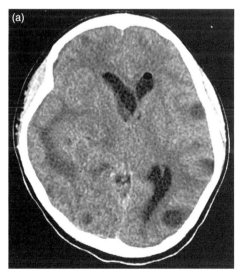 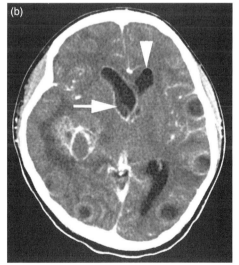

Fig. 17.3. Axial CT images: (a) pre- and (b) post-contrast, demonstrating multiple low-attenuation ring-enhancing lesions. Note the high-attenuation material within the right frontal horn (arrow) and a gas locule within the left frontal horn (arrowhead); ependymal enhancement is seen in the right lateral ventricle. The overall appearance is in keeping with multiple cerebral abscesses.

Chapter

18

Cervical spine

Characteristics

- The highest proportion of cervical spine injuries result from road traffic collisions.

- Falls from a height and sporting accidents make up the next largest categories.

- 50% of cervical spine injuries occur at C6 or C7.

- 33% of cervical spine injuries occur at C2.

- Cross-sectional imaging is performed when:
  - plain films are inadequate
  - if the cervical spine cannot be cleared clinically
  - when there has been a significant mechanism of injury

- Advancement and ease of access to CT has resulted in cross-sectional imaging being performed more frequently for cervical spine injuries.

- The aim of imaging is to identify an underlying injury, and to determine whether an injury is stable or unstable. Stability determines the management of the injury.

- Local guidance will determine scan protocols. The scan should typically extend from the base of the skull to T4, and images should be reviewed axially in conjunction with sagittal and coronal reformats. Correlation with clinical history can add important information and help to identify an abnormality.

- The spinal column maintains its stability through a complex network of ligaments. In order to assess stability, the spine is divided into three distinct columns: anterior, middle and posterior.
  - *Anterior column* contains the anterior longitudinal ligament and the anterior two-thirds of the vertebral bodies, annulus fibrosus and intervertebral discs.
  - *Middle column* contains the posterior longitudinal ligament and the posterior third of the vertebral bodies, annulus and intervertebral discs.
  - *Posterior column* contains the bony elements formed by the pedicles, transverse processes, articulating facets, laminae, and spinous processes.

- When one column is disrupted, the remaining two columns can provide sufficient stability to prevent spinal cord injury.

- When two or more columns are disrupted, the spinal column is regarded as unstable, as the spine can move as separate units, increasing the occurrence of spinal cord injury.

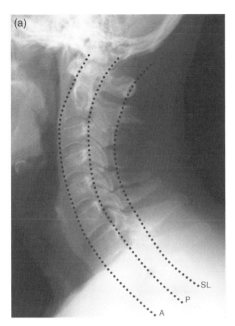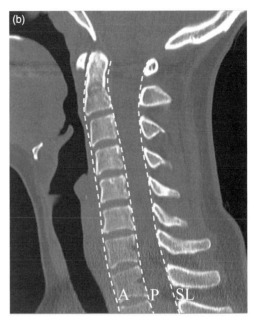

Fig. 18.1. (a) Normal lateral radiography and (b) normal mid-sagittal CT cervical spine with three lines: anterior vertebral (A), posterior vertebral (P) and spinolaminar (SP), showing normal alignment.

'ABCS' approach to interpreting multiplanar reformats of the CT cervical spine

A Alignment

- Normal articulation of the craniocervical junction should be assessed on the sagittal and axial planes; subluxation usually results from ligamentous injury.

- Normal smooth curves of the anterior vertebral, posterior vertebral and spinolaminar lines should be identified on the sagittal reconstruction, similar to the interpretation of a lateral cervical spine radiograph (Fig. 18.1).

- In a child, pseudo-subluxation of C2 on C3 may be identified, which can cause confusion. In these cases, examine the spinolaminar line from C1 to C3 on sagittal reconstructions. If the bases of the spinous processes lie >2 mm from this line, an injury should be suspected. Correlate with soft-tissue findings (see below).

- The distance between the anterior arch of C1 and the odontoid peg (the predental space) should be <3 mm in an adult and <5 mm in a child, measured on the mid-sagittal image, similar to the criteria used on a lateral radiograph.

- Facet joint alignment should be assessed on the axial and sagittal images. The *hamburger sign* confirms normal alignment of the facet joint on axial images, with the two halves of the 'burger bun' contributed to by the superior and inferior articular facets. In facet dislocation, the *reverse hamburger sign* is described, where the orientation of the 'burger bun' halves is reversed; the dislocation is apparent in the sagittal plane.

- The tips of the spinous processes should align in the midline in the coronal plane, similar to their appearance on an AP (anteroposterior) radiograph. Bifid spinous processes can make interpretation difficult.

B Bone
- Vertebral bodies should be of uniform height, best assessed in the sagittal and coronal planes. Increase in density or loss of vertebral height is in keeping with a compression fracture. Retropulsion of a fracture fragment into the spinal canal may result in spinal cord compression.
- Assess for the normal bony cortical outline. A breach in the cortex suggests a fracture; however, vascular channels also appear as lucent lines reaching the cortex and can be misinterpreted as a fracture. Correlation of these lines in all three planes helps to confirm the actual presence of a fracture.

C Cartilage
- The intervertebral spaces should be of uniform height in both the sagittal and coronal planes.
- Widening of the intervertebral spaces, or interspinous distances, may indicate an unstable dislocation.
- An increase in the interspinous distance of more than 50% suggests ligamentous disruption. Muscular spasm can make interpretation difficult.

S Soft tissues
- Retropharyngeal soft-tissue swelling may be the only sign of a significant injury; swelling takes time to form and may not be apparent if imaging is performed too early post injury.
- Normal retropharyngeal measurements are <7 mm anterior to C2–C4 (one-third of a vertebral body width at this level), and <22 mm below C5 (one vertebral body width).
- Judicial assessment of the structures surrounding the cervical spine is important in order to identify associated injuries. Examples include: mandibular fractures, temporomandibular joint subluxation/dislocation, injury to the aerodigestive tract, pneumomediastinum, fractures of ribs/sternum/scapula, and pneumothorax. This list is not exhaustive and careful interpretation is essential to ensure that significant injuries are not missed.
- Most importantly, where spinal cord or ligamentous injury is suspected, MRI should be performed to assess further.
- Cervical spine injuries can be classified according to the mechanism of injury (Fig. 18.2). These include flexion, flexion/rotation, extension, vertical compression and upper cervical spine injuries.

Tables 18.1–18.5 classify the types of cervical spine injuries, their radiological features and stability.

Table 18.1 Flexion injuries.

Fracture type	Description and radiological features	Stability
Simple wedge compression fracture	Compression fracture of the anterosuperior aspect of the vertebral body (Fig. 18.2) Prevertebral soft-tissue swelling. Reduced vertebral height anteriorly with increased concavity and sclerosis (secondary to impaction).	Stable unless associated with posterior ligamentous disruption (Fig. 18.3)
Flexion teardrop fracture (Fig. 18.4)	Flexion injury with vertical axial compression. Fracture through the antero-inferior aspect of the vertebral body, often with anterior displacement of the fragment ('teardrop'). Associated with significant ligamentous disruption. All three columns are disrupted. Associated with spinal cord injury. Differs from an extension teardrop fracture in that the anterior height of the vertebral body is usually reduced.	Unstable
Clay shoveller's fracture (Fig. 18.5)	Forced abrupt hyperflexion injury with neck and upper thoracic muscular contraction. Also caused by direct blow to the spinous processes. Commonly occurs in the lower cervical/upper thoracic spine. Oblique fracture of the base of a spinous process – avulsed by the supraspinous ligament. Vertical split appearance of the spinous process on AP (anteroposterior) view.	Stable
Anterior subluxation	Posterior ligamentous complex ruptures and the anterior longitudinal ligament remains intact. No associated bony injury. Sagittal view – widening of interspinous distance. Anterior and posterior lines are disrupted in flexion views.	Stable
Bilateral facet dislocation	Severe flexion injury from a large force. The vertebral body above displaces anteriorly by at least 50% of the AP diameter of the vertebral body. The inferior articulating facets of the upper vertebral body move superior and anterior to the superior articulating facets of the vertebral body below. The facets often appear 'locked'. Associated with disc herniation.	Highly unstable
Odontoid fracture (Fig. 18.6)	Type 1 occurs at the tip at the site of insertion of the alar ligament. Type 2 involves the junction with the body of C2. Most common type of odontoid fracture. Associated with non-union due to limited blood supply and small area of cancellous bone (Fig. 18.7). Type 3 extends into the body of C2 (Fig. 18.8).	Type 1 – stable Type 2 – unstable Type 3 – unstable if fragment separation
Uncinate process fracture	Lateral flexion injury.	Stable

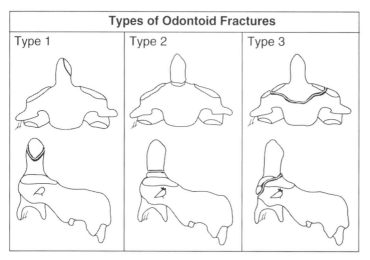

Fig. 18.6. Diagram showing types of odontoid peg fractures. Classification of odontoid peg fractures. From: *Sports Medicines: Problems and Practical Management* (Eds E. Sherry & D. Bokor); Greenwich Medical Media, 1997: page 117.

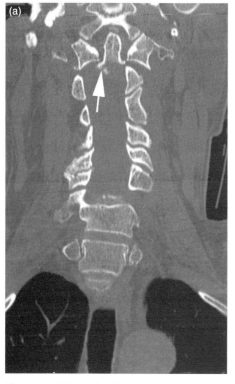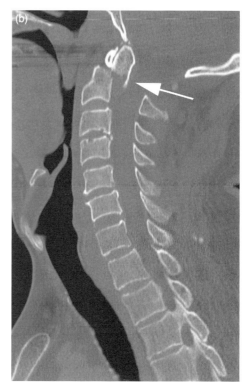

Fig. 18.7. (a) Coronal and (b) sagittal CT images demonstrating type 2 odontoid peg fracture (arrows).

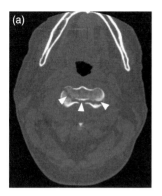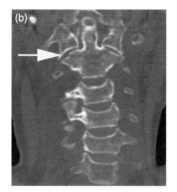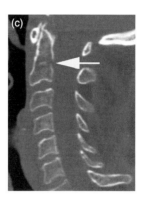

Fig. 18.8. (a) Axial (arrowheads), (b) coronal and (c) sagittal CT images (arrows) demonstrating a type 3 odontoid peg fracture.

Table 18.2 Rotational injuries.

Fracture type	Description and radiological features	Stability
Unilateral facet dislocation (Fig. 18.9)	Flexion/rotation injury. One inferior articular facet of an upper vertebral body passes superior and anterior to the superior articular facet of the vertebral body below and comes to rest in the intervertebral foramen. The vertebral body above displaces anteriorly by less than 50% of the AP diameter of the vertebral body (compare with bilateral facet dislocation). Coronal view – disruption of the line joining the spinous processes at the level of the dislocation. Oblique view – Disruption of the typical shingles appearance at the level of the dislocation.	Considered a stable injury unless it occurs at the C1/C2 level

Table 18.3 Extension injuries.

Fracture type	Description and radiological features	Stability
Fracture of posterior arch of the atlas	Hyperextension results in a compressive force which compresses the posterior neural arch of the atlas between the occiput and the dens. *Sagittal view* – fracture line through the posterior neural arch. *Coronal view* – fails to show displacement of the lateral masses of C1 with respect to the articular pillars of C2 (thus distinguishing this fracture from a Jefferson fracture).	Stable
Extension teardrop fracture	Common in diving injuries and usually occurs at C5–C7. True avulsion injury with the anterior longitudinal ligament avulsing the antero-inferior corner of the vertebral body. Vertebral body height is preserved. May be associated with central cord syndrome with buckling of the ligamentum flavum.	Highly unstable
Hangman's fracture (Fig. 18.10)	Traumatic bilateral fractures through the pedicles of C2 resulting in spondylolisthesis. Common in road traffic accidents. Fatal hangings result from a hyoid fracture and asphyxiation. There is disruption of the spinolaminar line.	Unstable

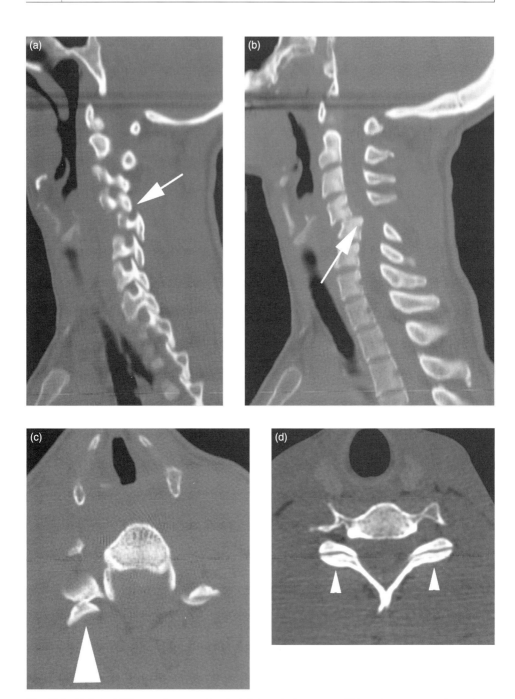

Fig. 18.9. (a) Sagittal CT image demonstrating the inferior articular process of C4 passing anterosuperior to the superior articular facet of C5 (arrow). (b) Sagittal CT image showing loss of anterior and posterior vertebral alignment and posterior displacement of C5 into the spinal canal (arrow). (c) Axial CT image demonstrating the *reverse hamburger sign*, in facet dislocation (arrowhead); compare with (d) normal axial facet alignment (arrowheads).

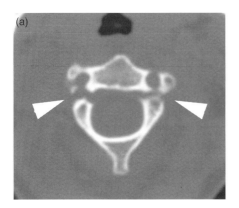

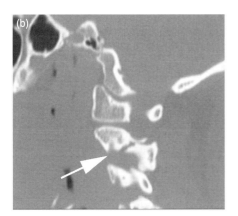

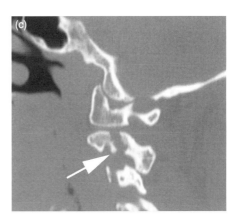

Fig. 18.10. (a) Axial (arrowheads) and (b), (c) sagittal CT images (arrows) demonstrating fractures through the pedicles of C2 bilaterally in keeping with hangman's fracture.

Table 18.4 Vertebral compression injuries.

Fracture type	Description and radiological features	Stability
Jefferson fracture (Fig. 18.11)	Burst fracture of the ring of C1 A compressive force is transmitted evenly through the occipital condyles to the superior articular surfaces of the lateral masses of C1. The masses are forced laterally, causing fractures of the anterior and posterior arches. There is usually disruption of the transverse ligament. **Sagittal view** – significant soft-tissue swelling. **Coronal odontoid view** – unilateral or bilateral displacement of the lateral masses of C1 with respect to the articular pillars of C2.	Unstable
Burst fracture	A downward compressive force is transmitted to lower vertebral bodies. The intervertebral disc is driven into the vertebral body below, causing it to shatter outwards. Both anterior and middle columns are disrupted. Comminuted vertebral body fracture with anterior and posterior displacement of fragments. Fracture fragments may impinge on the cord, causing anterior cord syndrome.	Unstable

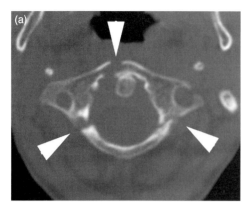
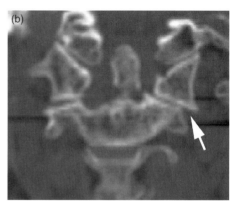

Fig. 18.11. (a) Axial CT image demonstrating burst fractures affecting the anterior and posterior arches of C1 in keeping with a Jefferson burst fracture (arrowheads). (b) Coronal CT image demonstrating lateral displacement of the C1 lateral mass (arrow), similar to the appearances of a Jefferson burst fracture on the 'peg' view of C spine radiograph series. There is also a concurrent fracture of the odontoid peg.

Table 18.5 Upper cervical spine injuries.

Fracture	Description and radiological features	Stability
Atlanto-occipital dislocation	Severe flexion or extension at the upper cervical level. Involves complete disruption of all ligamentous relationships between the occiput and the atlas. Death is often immediate due to stretching of the brainstem, causing respiratory arrest. There is disassociation between the base of the occiput and the arch of C1.	Highly unstable
Atlanto-axial subluxation	Flexion injury without a lateral or rotatory component at the upper cervical level. There is disruption of the transverse ligament. There are shearing forces, as the skull grinds the atlanto-axial complex in flexion. Neurologic injury may occur from cord compression between the odontoid and posterior arch of C1. Sagittal view – predentate space >3 mm in adults (>5 mm in children).	Highly unstable

Chapter

19

Neck vessel dissection

Characteristics

- Dissection is defined as elevation or separation of arterial wall layers, most commonly the intima, from the underlying media.

- Begins as a tear in the arterial wall allowing flowing blood, under arterial pressure, to enter and separate the layers, thus creating a false lumen. This results in potential ischaemia from arterial stenosis or occlusion.

- The resulting intimal haematoma, with or without aneurysm formation, is a source of micro-emboli and can lead to further cerebral ischaemia.

- Accounts for up to 25% of strokes in patients <50 years of age.

- Arterial dissection most commonly involves the carotid artery, and may affect both the extracranial and intracranial portions; the latter is more commonly involved, and often occurs just cranial to the bifurcation. Vertebral artery dissection occurs less frequently, and most commonly involves the extra-osseous segment at the C1–C2 level.

- Preceding trauma is common, and may be trivial, although spontaneous dissection can also occur. Other risk factors include hypertension and genetically related connective tissue disorders (Marfan syndrome, Ehlers–Danlos syndrome type IV and fibromuscular dysplasia). These may play a greater role in cases of minor trauma.

Clinical features

- Presentation may be non-specific and a high index of suspicion is critical.

- Severe constant head, neck and facial pain are common (75%).

- Partial Horner syndrome (miosis, enopthalmus and ptosis) is reported in carotid dissection.

- The majority (93%) of patients will have focal neurological deficit related to an ischaemic stroke at the time of diagnosis; this can be delayed for several weeks in extracranial dissection.

- Other signs of maxillofacial trauma, cervical spine injury, hanging or strangulation should alert clinicians to this associated injury.

Radiological features

CT angiography

- CT angiography is sensitive and accurate for rapid and non-invasive diagnosis.
- 50 ml of iodinated contrast injected via a pump, at 3–5 ml/s, followed by 50 ml of normal saline. Coverage should be from the aortic arch to the circle of Willis; injection should be bolus timed with a region of interest over the aortic arch.
- Study should be reviewed in axial slices, with multiplanar reformats and maximum-intensity projections.

Features

- A thin low-density intraluminal intimal flap may be seen, separating the high-density contrast within the lumen (Fig. 19.1).
- Centric or eccentric narrowing of the lumen may be observed. Associated crescentic thickening of the arterial wall is consistent with intramural haematoma.
- An absence of high-density contrast within the lumen suggests thrombosis and complete occlusion.
- Narrowing or dilatation of the calibre of the arterial lumen may also be observed.
- A careful search for associated injuries should be performed.

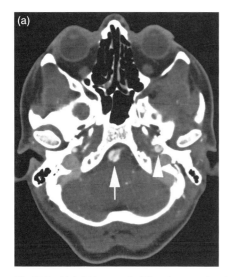 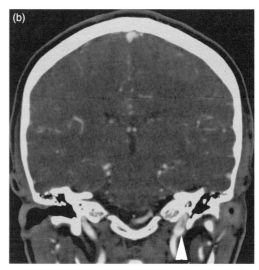

Fig 19.1. (a) Axial image of a CT angiogram, showing a dissection flap within the left internal carotid (arrowhead) and basilar (arrow) arteries. (b) Coronal image of a CT angiogram showing a left internal carotid artery dissection flap (arrowhead).

MRI/MR angiography

Features

- Absence of flow voids on conventional T2 spin echo sequences. High signal is seen within the affected vessels due to reduced blood flow/thrombosis (Fig. 19.2a). The low-signal-intensity intimal flap may also be seen (Fig. 19.2b).

- Mural haematoma may be seen, appearing as high signal in the vessel walls on T1W sequences.

- As in CT angiography, a dissection may be seen as a thin low-signal-intensity flap within gadolinium-enhanced vessels on MR angiography. Narrowing or calibre change may also be demonstrated, with the dissection sometimes described as the *MRA string sign*.

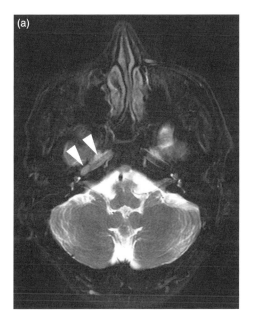 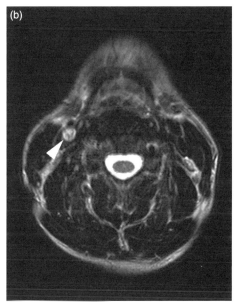

Fig. 19.2. Axial T2W MRI neck images: (a) high signal within the petrous portion of the right internal carotid secondary to absence of flow void/thrombosis (arrowheads); (b) dissection flap within a thrombosed right internal carotid artery (arrowhead).

Aortic dissection

Characteristics

- Life-threatening condition, with an incidence of 2 per 10,000. Most commonly seen in men aged 40–70 years (75%).

- Two to three times more common than aortic rupture, with 33% mortality within 24 hours if left untreated.

- Results from a tear in the intimal wall. Blood inflow at arterial pressure causes the formation of a subintimal haematoma and false lumen, by splitting the arterial wall in a longitudinal fashion.

- Involvement of the major branches arising from the aorta can occur, including abdominal arteries, resulting in reduced or occluded flow to major organs.

- Risk factors include hypertension, connective tissue disorders (Marfan syndrome, Ehlers–Danlos syndrome), aortic coarctation, bicuspid aortic valve, pregnancy, and collagen vascular disorders.

- Traumatic dissection occurs due to shearing forces from a decelerating injury. The dissection originates from a fixed point of the aorta, most commonly at the aortic isthmus, just distal to the left subclavian artery (i.e. at the ligamentum arteriosum). Other sites include the ascending aorta, the aortic root and at the diaphragmatic hiatus.

Clinical features

- An estimated 38% of dissections are missed on initial evaluation; therefore a high index of suspicion is vital.

- Up to 90% of patients report the sudden onset of chest pain, which can radiate to the neck (aortic arch) and back into the interscapular region (descending aorta).

- Neurological or stroke-like symptoms can occur, with involvement of the carotid or vertebral arteries.

- Myocardial infarction suggests involvement of the coronary ostia.

- Dyspnoea and orthopnoea may be reported if dissection ruptures into the pleural spaces.

- Blood pressure discrepancies between extremities may be seen, suggesting involvement of the limb arteries.

Radiological features

CT

- Pre-contrast study followed by CT angiography: 100 ml of iodinated contrast via pump injection at 3–5 ml/s with coverage from the aortic arch to the iliac arteries. Arterial-phase bolus timing is achieved with a region of interest over the thoracic aorta.

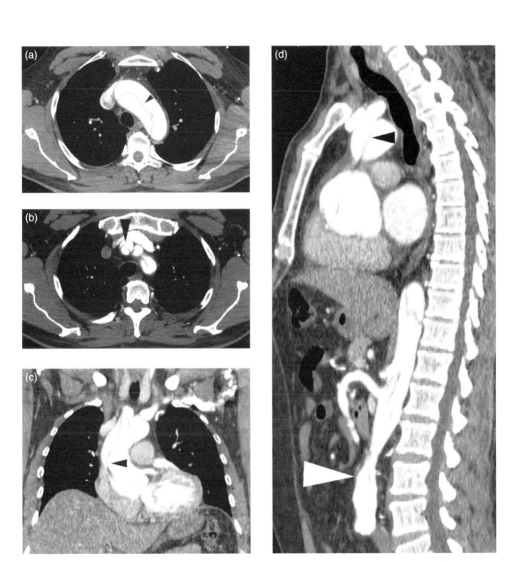

Fig. 20.1. Type A aortic dissection: (a) axial image demonstrating a thin low-attenuation dissection flap within the aortic arch (black arrowhead); (b) axial image demonstrating dissection flaps extending into the brachiocephalic (black arrowhead), left common carotid and left subclavian arteries; (c) coronal image demonstrating dissection flap originating from the aortic root (black arrowhead); (d) sagittal image demonstrating dissection flap extending from the ascending aorta (black arrowhead) into the abdominal aorta (white arrowhead).

- An electrocardiogram (ECG) gated study should be considered, where available, as pulsation artefacts from the heart and aortic root may lead to a false appearance of an intimal flap at the aortic root. Involvement of the coronary ostia may also be detected with ECG gated studies, which is particularly important in cases involving the ascending aorta.

- Study should be reviewed on axial slices, with multiplanar reformats and maximum-intensity projections.

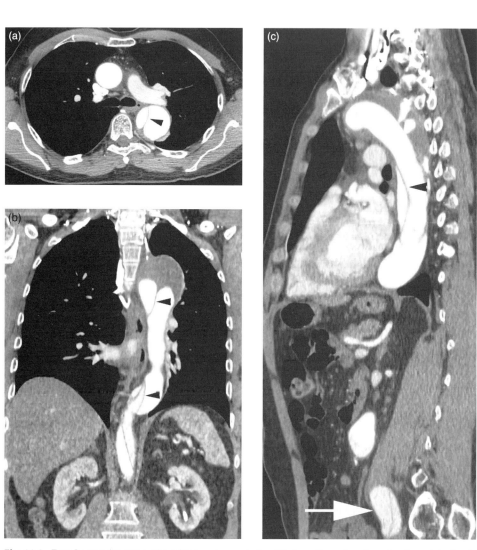

Fig. 20.2. Type B aortic dissection: (a) axial image demonstrating thin low-attenuation dissection flap originating in the descending thoracic aorta (black arrowhead); (b) coronal image demonstrating dissection flap originating from the descending aorta distal to the left subclavian artery origin (black arrowheads); (c) sagittal image demonstrating dissection flap extending from the descending aorta (black arrowhead) into the abdominal aorta (white arrow). Note also the increased attenuation of the mediastinal fat, consistent with haematoma.

Features

- High-density crescentic intramural haematoma is only evident in the pre-contrast phase, as the high-density intraluminal contrast in the angiographic phase will obscure this finding. Intramural haematoma may progress to frank dissection. Treatment is similar to that of a dissection in the same location.
- A thin low-density intraluminal intimal flap may be seen in up to 90% of cases, separating the high-density contrast within the lumen (Fig. 20.1).
- The origin of the dissection flap defines aortic dissection classification (Fig. 20.2), thereby determining management (Table 20.1).
- The true lumen is usually smaller with aortic wall calcification seen laterally. The false lumen is usually larger and has an irregular contour. Opacification is often delayed due to slower blood flow through the false channel.
- Periaortic or mediastinal haematoma appears as high-density stranding within normally low-density mediastinal fat.

Table 20.1 Classification of aortic dissection and optimal management.

DeBakey classification	Stanford classification	Management
I (50%): Ascending and descending aorta* II (10%): Ascending aorta only	A (60%): Involvement of ascending aorta	Surgery
III (40%): Limited to descending aorta*	B (40%): Limited to descending aorta*	Medical therapy with BP control: emerging role of endovascular stenting

*Descending aorta is defined as distal to the left subclavian artery origin.

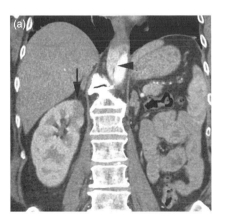 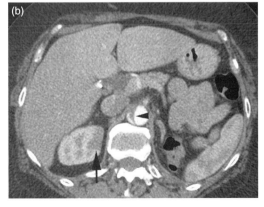

Fig. 20.3. (a) Axial and (b) coronal images demonstrating a wedge-shaped area of low attenuation within the upper pole of the right kidney, in keeping with infarction (black arrow). This is secondary to the dissection flap (black arrowhead) extending into the right renal artery.

- High-density fluid (>50 HU) may be seen within the pleural and pericardial spaces, indicating haematoma extension. The latter increases the risk of cardiac tamponade, aortic insufficiency and coronary artery involvement – all requiring urgent surgical management.
- Extension of the intimal flap may be seen within branch vessels. The absence of intraluminal contrast suggests vessel thrombosis, which may be secondary to false lumen formation.
- A delayed-phase study may demonstrate wedge-shaped low densities within the liver, spleen or kidneys, denoting areas of infarction (Fig. 20.3). Bowel-wall thickening, suggestive of bowel ischaemia, may be seen if mesenteric vessels are involved.

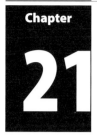

Chapter

21 Thoracic aortic aneurysm and rupture

Characteristics

- An aneurysm is defined as dilatation of the aorta >150% of its normal diameter. For the thoracic aorta, a diameter >3.5 cm is considered dilated and >4.5 cm aneurysmal.
- The incidence is 5.9 cases per 100,000 person-years, with most detected incidentally due to increasing use of imaging. 25% of patients may also have an associated abdominal aortic aneurysm.
- Rupture and dissection are commonly associated life-threatening complications, with a mortality of 3.5 per 100,000 persons.
- Atherosclerosis is the most common cause. Other risk factors include connective tissue disorders (Marfan and Ehlers–Danlos syndromes), syphilis, mycotic aneurysms, aortitis secondary to Takayasu's arteritis, giant cell aortitis and Kawasaki disease.
- True aneurysms involve all three layers of the vessel wall, and tend to be fusiform-shaped with circumferential symmetrical dilatation.
- Pseudoaneurysms involve, and are contained by, the outer adventitial layer of the vessel wall. These tend to be saccular, with a localized outpouching of the aortic wall, and are seen more commonly in post-traumatic, mycotic and post-surgical aneurysms.
- Rupture may occur in trauma, especially secondary to the deceleration shearing forces found in road traffic accidents, where the aortic isthmus is most commonly involved (95%). Only 15–20% of patients survive to reach the emergency department for further management. Ruptures in survivors are often contained by a pseudoaneurysm.

Clinical features

- Most patients with aneurysms are asymptomatic and incidentally diagnosed.
- Compressive symptoms may develop and are related to the structures involved:
  - Superior vena cava – distended neck veins
  - Recurrent laryngeal nerve – hoarse voice
  - Trachea and bronchus – dyspnoea, stridor, wheezing or coughing
  - Oesophagus – dysphagia
  - Spine/spinal cord/thrombosis of spinal arteries – neurological symptoms with paraparesis or paraplegia.

- Aneurysmal dilatation of the aortic root is specifically associated with aortic regurgitation, manifests as a cardiac murmur.
- Erosion into adjacent structures may present as haemoptysis, haematemesis and GI bleeding.
- Acute pain suggests imminent rupture or dissection, with the pattern of pain suggestive of the segment involved:
  o Ascending aorta – anterior chest pain
  o Aortic arch – neck pain
  o Descending aorta – interscapular or back pain
  o Diaphragmatic hiatus – mid-back and epigastric pain.

Radiological features

CT

- Presentation may be similar to an aortic dissection and hence a similar imaging protocol should be employed for both. A pre-contrast study followed by CT angiography should be performed.
- An ECG gated study should be considered where available.
- The study should be reviewed in axial slices with multiplanar reformats and maximum-intensity projections.
- Point-of-care ultrasound using a suprasternal window can be useful to confirm aortic dilatation.

Features

- Aneurysmal dilatation of the aorta can be readily assessed.
- Low-density crescentic mural thrombus is often seen within the aneurysm sac.
- Focal outpouching, consistent with a pseudoaneurysm, may be seen in a contained rupture (Fig. 21.1). Focal ectasia (point aneurysm) may be observed, suggesting impending rupture.
- High-density stranding or contrast extravasation within the pericardium and mediastinum confirms rupture (see Fig. 20.2c).
- Erosion, resulting in aortocaval and aortopulmonary fistulae, is delineated by the presence of high-density contrast contiguous with the aorta.
- High-density fluid (>50 HU) may be seen within the pleural space, suggesting a haemothorax.

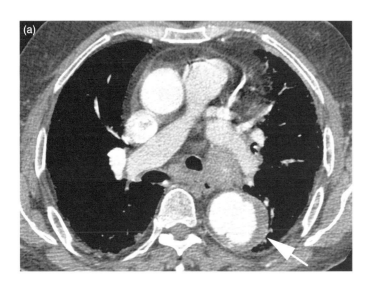

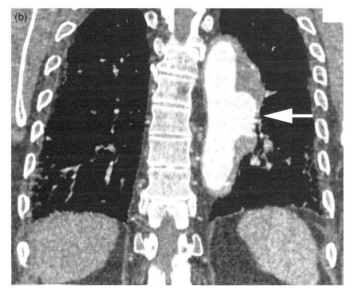

Fig 21.1. (a) Axial and (b) coronal image demonstrating outpouching of the descending thoracic aorta in keeping with a pseudoaneurysm (arrows).

Chapter

22

Diaphragmatic rupture

Characteristics

- A relatively rare diagnosis seen in ~5% of all patients with blunt trauma. May also result from a penetrating injury.
- 90% of cases are related to motor vehicle collisions, with a two-fold mechanism:
  - *Lateral impact*, causing distortion of the chest wall, leading to laceration in the central or posterior portion of the ipsilateral diaphragm.
  - *Frontal impact*, causing raised intra-abdominal pressure, leading to a radial tear in the embryological posterolateral weak point of the diaphragm.
- Apparent preponderance for the left diaphragm (80–90%); this was originally attributed to the protection of the right hemidiaphragm by the liver. Now thought to be related to the greater extent of injuries, and thus higher mortality, associated with right-sided trauma, which is therefore less commonly diagnosed.
- Penetrating injuries from gunshot and knife wounds to the chest and abdomen may injure the diaphragm. These are usually small and may present later, after years of gradual herniation and enlargement.

Clinical features

- Presentation may be non-specific, with respiratory symptoms such as dyspnoea being most common. A high index of suspicion is required.
- Mechanism of injury should trigger a search for a diaphragmatic rupture.
- Associated injuries include pelvic fractures (40%), splenic rupture (25%), liver laceration (25%) and thoracic aortic tears (5–10%).
- Diagnosis is often delayed, by months or years, with up to 50% undiagnosed in the first 24 hours.
- Auscultation of bowel sounds in the chest, or dullness to percussion, suggest herniation of intra-abdominal content into the thoracic cavity via a defect. Patients may also present late, with obstruction secondary to strangulation of the herniated bowel.

Radiological features

CT

- CT scan should be performed with intravenous (i.v.) and oral contrast. Visceral organs and bowel loops will enhance and herniated organs can be identified easily within the thorax.

Features

- Discontinuity of the hemidiaphragm may be observed, but breathing artefacts may cause false positives as patients are often dyspnoeic.
- The stomach and colon are the most common organs to herniate on the left, and the liver on the right.
- The *dependent viscera sign* results from the lack of posterior diaphragmatic support of the adjacent abdominal viscera due to diaphragmatic rupture. This sign is present when the upper third of the liver abuts the posterior ribs on the right side, or the stomach, spleen or bowel abuts the posterior ribs on the left side (Fig. 22.1a, b).
- The *collar sign* denotes a waist-like constriction of a herniated viscus at the level of the diaphragmatic tear. This is more easily appreciated on the left, while indentation in the liver is more difficult to appreciate in a right-sided injury (Fig. 22.1c, d).
- These findings are often best appreciated on multiplanar reformats, where the extent of the injury can be assessed in order to aid surgical management.
- A careful search for other injuries is vital, as diaphragmatic injuries rarely occur in isolation.

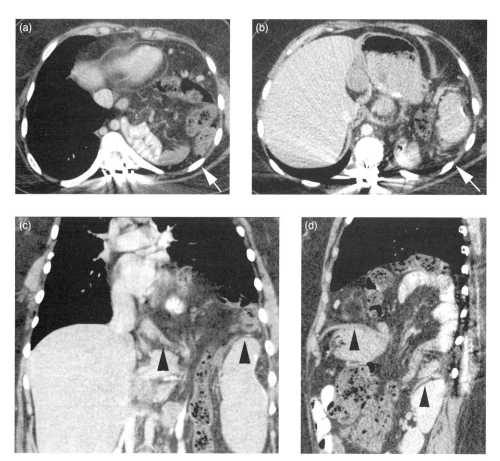

Fig. 22.1. Diaphragmatic rupture: (a), (b) axial images demonstrating bowel and intra-abdominal fat lying anterior to the posterior ribs (arrow), in keeping with the *dependent viscera sign*; (c) coronal and (d) sagittal images demonstrating discontinuity of diaphragmatic slips (arrowheads) and herniation of abdominal content through the defect in the diaphragm, in keeping with the *collar sign*.

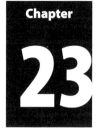

Chapter

23

Haemothorax

Characteristics

- Defined as the accumulation of blood in the pleural cavity. A relatively common problem resulting from injury to intrathoracic structures, pleura or the chest wall.

- Most common cause is trauma, including both penetrating and blunt trauma.

- Other less common, non-trauma-related, aetiologies include neoplasia, blood dyscrasias, pulmonary emboli, tuberculosis, arteriovenous fistulae, hereditary haemorrhagic telangiectasia, great vessel aneurysms, and abdominal pathologies such as pancreatitis and haemoperitoneum.

- The progressive lysis of red cells within a haemothorax leads to increased protein content of the effusion. This creates an osmotic gradient encouraging transudation of the intravascular fluid. A previously small-volume haemothorax can progress into a larger-volume effusion and cause symptoms.

- Additional complications of haemothorax include:
  - *Empyema* – bacterial contamination and growth
  - *Fibrothorax* – fibrin deposition coating the visceral and parietal pleural layers, preventing lung expansion and reducing lung function.

Clinical features

- Haemothoraces rarely occur in isolation and patients will often be symptomatic from the additional intrathoracic or chest wall injuries.

- Can be divided into haemodynamic and respiratory effects.
  - *Haemodynamic* – cardiovascular instability results primarily from vascular blood loss. This can be compounded by cardiac dysfunction and multifactorial coagulopathy in trauma.
  - *Respiratory* – the collection exerts a space-occupying effect preventing normal ventilation, producing symptoms of dyspnoea. This may progress slowly in non-traumatic cases. Pain and mechanical chest wall disruption will further limit respiratory efficacy.

- Reduced air entry and dullness to percussion will be detected with large-volume collections. This may be difficult to assess in the trauma situation, where the patient is supine and the effusion layers posteriorly.

Radiological features

Ultrasound

Features

- eFAST (extended Focused Assessment Sonography in Trauma) is often used in the trauma setting to detect the presence of free fluid within the abdomen and chest. Views of the upper quadrants of the abdomen are obtained routinely to assess for sub-diaphragmatic free fluid.

- An anechoic (black) collection lying superior to the echogenic diaphragm is consistent with pleural fluid (Fig. 23.1).

- Ultrasound is able to detect an effusion as small as 20 ml.

- As clotting occurs, the collection become hypoechoic rather than uniformly anechoic.

- Careful observation during breathing will demonstrate a swirling movement pattern with an evolving haemothorax.

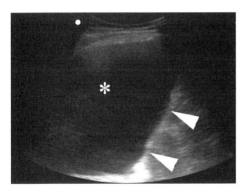

Fig. 23.1. Ultrasound image demonstrating a large left-sided, predominantly anechoic, fluid collection (asterix) lying above the diaphragm (white arrowheads), containing scattered dependent internal echoes. The appearance is in keeping with a left haemothorax.

CT

Features

- Crescentic, lenticular or elliptical low density, lying in a dependent position, confirms the presence of pleural fluid.

- Haemothorax is suggested when the density of this fluid measures >50 HU. With progressive clotting, a layering effect may become apparent, where the denser clot/blood gravitates to a dependent position, while the remaining fluid in the collection persists in a non-dependent position (Fig. 23.2).

- Active extravasation of contrast from a traumatized vessel may be seen extending into the pleural fluid. A swirling pattern of contrast may be observed within the collection, or the overall density of the collection may increase.

- A careful search for an associated vascular or chest wall injury is necessary. In cases where a thoracic injury is not demonstrated, the pathology may relate to injury of an abdominal organ, such as laceration of a solid viscus.

- Complications of a haemothorax usually occur following a delay from the time of the initial injury.

  - An empyema appears as a loculated collection, containing multiple septations, developing within the low-density collection. The adjacent pleura is thickened and enhances post contrast (Fig. 23.3). Ultrasound is more sensitive than CT in identifying small septations within the empyema (Fig. 23.4).

  - Calcification and pleural thickening are observed in cases of fibrothorax, although this only becomes apparent following a long delay after the initial injury.

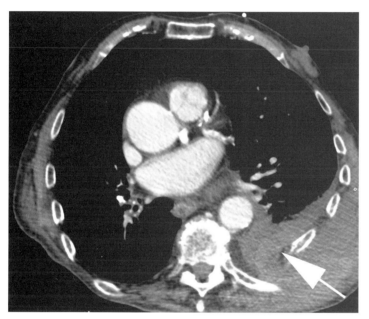

Fig. 23.2. Axial image demonstrating high-attenuation fluid layering posteriorly within the collection in keeping with a haemothorax (arrow).

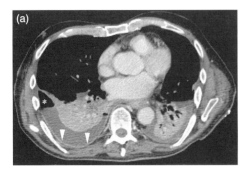

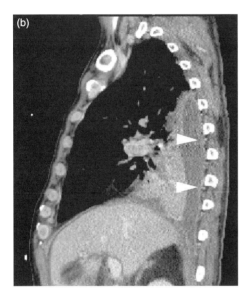

Fig. 23.3. (a) Axial and (b) sagittal images demonstrating a gas-containing right pleural collection (asterix) with a thickened enhanced pleura (arrowheads), consistent with an empyema. There is also a small left-sided pleural effusion and bilateral lower lobe consolidation.

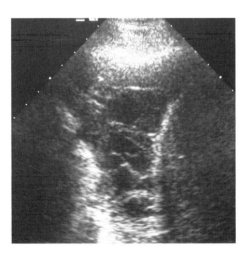

Fig. 23.4. Ultrasound image demonstrating a heavily septated collection in keeping with an empyema.

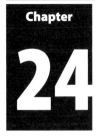

Chapter

24

Oesophageal perforation

Characteristics

- Oesophageal perforation is a medical emergency.
- The oesophagus lacks a serosal layer, unlike the rest of the alimentary tract, and is consequently more vulnerable to injury.
- The loose surrounding stromal connective tissue of the oesophagus permits the rapid spread of infection and inflammation through the tissue planes into surrounding structures, resulting in sepsis.
- Iatrogenic causes account for up to 85% of perforations. They are most commonly related to endoscopic interventions such as dilatation of achalasia or malignant strictures. Intra-operative injury, related to cardiothoracic surgery or fundoplication, accounts for approximately 2% of cases.
- The rare and dangerous entity of spontaneous perforation, also known as *Boerhaave's syndrome*, accounts for 15% of cases. Perforation results from an abrupt increase in intra-abdominal pressure during vomiting against a closed superior oesophageal sphincter.
- Other rarer causes include the ingestion of caustic substances and foreign bodies, and trauma. Penetrating trauma most commonly affects the cervical oesophagus.
- Morbidity results from leakage of the gastric contents into the mediastinal and pleural spaces. This causes an inflammatory response leading to mediastinitis, pneumonia, empyema and sepsis. Mortality is most commonly associated with Boerhaave's syndrome, due to a delay in making the initial diagnosis.

Clinical features

- Iatrogenic injury is usually identified during the procedure. Alternatively, patients may complain of neck or chest pain, dysphagia, odynophagia, dyspnoea and symptoms of sepsis following an endoscopic procedure.
- Patients with Boerhaave's syndrome typically present with the *Mackler triad* of vomiting, chest pain and subcutaneous emphysema.
- Features of sepsis, namely tachypnoea, tachycardia, hypotension and fever, are common initial findings.

- *Hamman's sign* describes the 'crunching' sound heard over the precordium with each heartbeat in the presence of a pneumomediastinum, which can be associated with oesophageal perforation.
- Reduced breath sounds and dullness to percussion suggest the presence of a pleural effusion secondary to gastric content leakage into the pleural cavity.

Radiological features

CT

- The study should be acquired following intravenous (i.v.) contrast with coverage to include the neck, chest and upper abdomen, in order to ensure that the whole oesophagus has been included.
- Water-soluble oral contrast can be given just before the patient is put onto the scan table.

Features (Fig. 24.1)

- The oesophageal wall is usually thickened.
- High-density stranding within the (normally low-density) mediastinal fat suggests mediastinitis. Extraluminal mediastinal contrast may be demonstrated, confirming the perforation. The location of this may help to identify the site of perforation.
- Reviewing images on lung windows will aid in the detection of extraluminal gas within the mediastinum, usually adjacent to the site of perforation. This may extend into the pleural cavity to produce a pneumothorax or, more commonly,

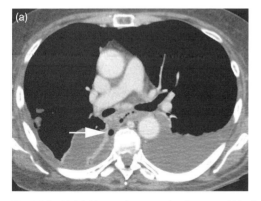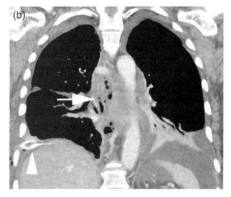

Fig. 24.1. (a) Axial image demonstrating free gas within the mediastinum. There are several tiny locules of gas adjacent to the oesophagus at the level of the perforation (arrow), and bilateral pleural effusions. (b) Coronal image demonstrating a pneumomediastinum secondary to oesophageal perforation (arrow). There are bilateral pleural effusions, left basal consolidation and ascites. A right chest drain is in situ (arrowhead)

dissect into the neck and soft-tissue planes of the chest wall, resulting in subcutaneous emphysema.

- A low-density crescentic dependent collection within the pleural cavity usually represents an effusion secondary to gastric content leakage. An empyema may develop with time, and is demonstrated by enhancement and thickening of the adjacent pleura.

Chapter

25

Pericardial effusion/cardiac tamponade

Characteristics

- The pericardium consists of visceral and parietal layers, which envelop the four cardiac chambers and origin of the great vessels.
- These two layers are lubricated by a small volume (15–50 ml) of serous fluid resulting from an ultrafiltrate of plasma.
- The pericardium and pericardial fluid are important in normal cardiac functions as they:
  - ○ Contribute to resting diastolic pressure
  - ○ Ensure uniform contraction of the myocardium
  - ○ Limit excessive dilatation of the chambers in a hypervolaemic state.
- The pericardium accommodates fluctuations in pericardial fluid volume by increasing the pericardial compliance. This lessens the increase in intrapericardial pressure.
- *Cardiac tamponade* results in an increase in intrapericardial pressure, causing haemodynamic compromise. Initially this limits diastolic filling, progressing to impairment of all cardiac chambers throughout the cardiac cycle.
- Existing medical problems cause approximately 60% of pericardial effusions, and relate to the obstruction of venous or lymphatic drainage from the heart. Common causes include heart failure, renal insufficiency, infection (bacterial, viral or TB), neoplasia (lung – particularly mesothelioma, breast, lymphoma) or injury (iatrogenic, trauma, aortic dissection or myocardial infarction).

Clinical features

- Symptoms are dependent on the rate of fluid accumulation. Rapid elevation to as little as 80 ml may cause raised intrapericardial pressure and induce symptoms. Chronic gradual elevation with adaptation of myocardial compliance may not cause symptoms.
- Common symptoms include dyspnoea, chest discomfort, pericardial pain, dizziness and coughing.
- Specific signs of cardiac tamponade include diminished heart sounds, pericardial friction rub and features of hypotension (cold, clammy skin and weak pulse).
- Other classic descriptions include:
  - ○ *Beck's triad* – elevated jugular venous pressure (JVP) hypotension and diminished heart sounds

- o *Pulsus paradoxus* – exaggeration (>12 mmHg or 9%) of the normal inspiratory decrease in systemic blood pressure
- o *Kussmaul sign* – most commonly associated with constrictive pericarditis; describes paradoxical increase in venous distension during inspiration
- o *Ewart sign* – (also known as *Pins sign*) – area of dullness, with bronchial breath sounds, below the angle of the left scapula secondary to pericardial effusion.

Radiological features

Ultrasound

Features

- The subxyphoid window pericardial view is utilized in FAST (Focused Assessment Sonography in Trauma) to assess for pericardial effusions in trauma. Left parasternal long- and short-axis views are useful to assess for functional compromise.
- Care must be taken not to misinterpret a pleural effusion as a pericardial effusion.
- An anechoic/hypoechoic fluid collection is seen surrounding the heart, bounded by the pericardium (Fig. 25.1). The echogenicity of the collection increases if the effusion is associated with infection or the presence of blood/haematoma. With progressive increase in the depth of pericardial fluid >1 cm, compression of the cardiac chambers may be demonstrated, confirming cardiac tamponade. This affects the right atrium (RA) and right ventricle (RV) first, followed by the left atrium (LA) and last – and rarely – the left ventricle (LV).
- Fine septated loculations within the effusion suggest an infective cause, which is difficult to detect on CT.
- Ultrasound-guided pericardiocentesis increases procedural safety and success, compared with the traditional technique using anatomical landmarks.

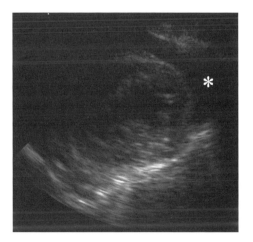

Fig. 25.1. Ultrasound image demonstrating large anechoic collection (asterix) surrounding the cardiac chambers in keeping with pericardial effusion.

CT

Features

- Studies are performed with i.v. contrast to aid demonstration of the pericardium and/or pericardial enhancement seen in infection/infiltration.
- A pericardial effusion as small as 20 ml can be detected on CT.
- Fluid typically accumulates in the dependent portion, posterior to the left ventricle, and appears as a low-density crescentic collection bound by the pericardium.
- With a progressive increase in volume, the effusion will expand lateral and anterior to the right atrium and right ventricle. Further increase will see an extension of the effusion into the superior pericardial recess. Large effusions will appear as a concentric low-density collection encircling the heart (Fig. 25.2).
- The density of the collection may help to identify the underlying pathology. Simple effusions have a density similar to water (0–10 HU), while an increase in density may be due to the presence of blood, pus or malignant infiltration.
- Pericardial thickening of >2 mm or the presence of loculations within the fluid suggests an infective cause for the effusion. Pericardial enhancement may also be seen in association with infection.
- A careful search for the underlying cause of the pericardial effusion is essential to aid management.
- With progressive enlargement of the effusion, compression of the adjacent cardiac chamber may become evident, suggesting development of a cardiac tamponade (Fig. 25.3).

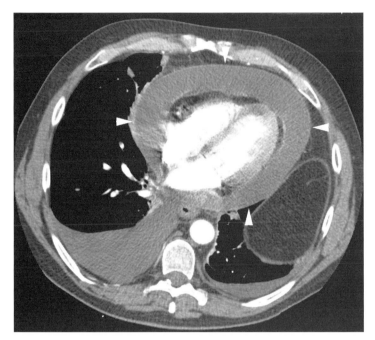

Fig.25.2. Axial image demonstrating a large low-density collection pericardial effusion encircling the heart (arrowheads), and bilateral pleural effusions.

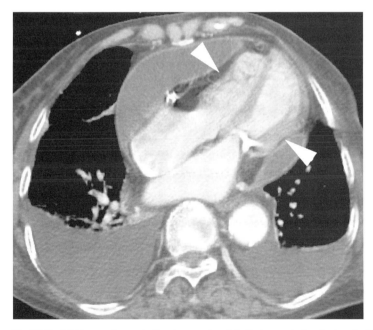

Fig.25.3. Axial image demonstrating large pericardial effusion encircling the heart with compression of the ventricles (arrowheads); bilateral pleural effusions are present.

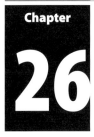

Chapter

26

Pneumothorax

Characteristics

- Pneumothorax is defined as the presence of gas within the pleural cavity, a potential space between the visceral and parietal pleura of the lung.
- Causes are divided into several categories.
  - *Primary spontaneous* – occurs in patients without underlying lung disease and in the absence of any preceding trauma. Most commonly seen in tall young people; thought to be related to increased shear forces at the lung apices. Other risk factors include smoking, Marfan syndrome and pregnancy.
  - *Secondary* – related to a variety of parenchymal lung diseases including chronic obstructive pulmonary disease (COPD), asthma, bronchogenic carcinoma, metastatic malignancy (sarcoma, genito-urinary tumour), TB, cystic fibrosis, interstitial lung disease, pulmonary fibrosis and acute respiratory distress syndrome (ARDS). Catamenial pneumothorax occurs secondary to endometriosis involving the diaphragm, usually within 72 hours of menstruating.
  - *Iatrogenic* – incidence is 5–7 per 10,000 hospital admissions following procedures such as transbronchial or transthoracic biopsy, central line insertion and positive pressure ventilation.
  - *Traumatic* – Penetrating injuries and blunt force trauma.
- With progressive air trapping within the pleural space, a tension pneumothorax ensues; the rising positive pressure compresses the great vessels within the mediastinum and diminishes venous return, reducing cardiac output and resulting in shock.
- The ipsilateral lung collapses under the positive pressure, impairing gaseous exchange, resulting in hypoxaemia.
- Tension pneumothorax most commonly occurs both in the setting of trauma, where the wound creates a one-way valve effect into the pleural space, and in the setting of positive pressure ventilation in intensive-care patients.

Clinical features

- Typical presentation in the majority of patients is an acute onset of pleuritic chest pain with dyspnoea. Non-specific symptoms including cough and malaise can also be present.

- Features associated with underlying lung disease may be present.
- Clinical history may suggest iatrogenic or traumatic causes.
- Asymmetric chest wall expansion, hyper-resonance and reduced/absent breath sounds are common findings.
- In tension pneumothorax, clinical examination may reveal tachypnoea, tachycardia, hypotension, raised JVP, and pulsus paradoxus.
- Early diagnosis in patients on positive pressure ventilation is vital, as rapid expansion of the pneumothorax will develop secondary to the positive pressure. Urgent treatment is particularly important in these patients who may have pre-existing reduced lung function due to co-morbidities.

Radiological features

Ultrasound

Features

- Useful in the setting of trauma, where supine chest radiographs are taken and an anterior pneumothorax may be difficult to appreciate.
- A high-frequency (5–12 MHz) linear probe is used to image the intercostal space.
- The pleura normally appears echogenic on ultrasound (Fig. 26.1a), and sliding of the visceral pleura is demonstrated on dynamic examination, referred to as the *lung sliding sign*.
- This sliding motion is absent in pneumothorax, as the gas collection within the pleural space displaces the visceral pleura away from the parietal pleura adherent to the chest wall.
- In the presence of a pneumothorax, reverberation artefacts (multiple equidistant echogenic lines) are demonstrated beneath the pleural layer (Fig. 26.2a).
- Mapping of the pneumothorax is possible by examination of the anterior and lateral chest wall. The *lung point* is described as the level at which pleural sliding is again seen, representing the margin of the pneumothorax.
- M-mode ultrasound is extremely useful. Normal lung pattern is described by the *sea shore sign* (Fig. 26.1b), while a pneumothorax has a different appearance on M-mode referred to as the *bar code* or *stratosphere sign* (Fig. 26.2b).

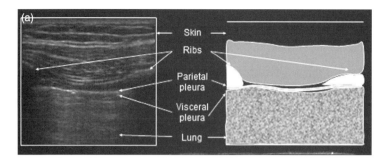

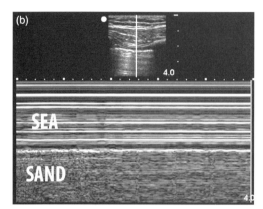

Fig. 26.1. Ultrasound images: (a) B-mode image normal lung, with line drawing demonstrating the separate structures; (b) M-mode image of normal lung demonstrating the *sea shore sign*.

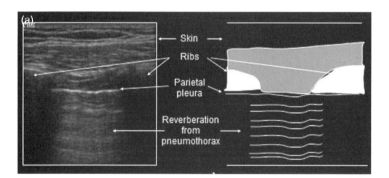

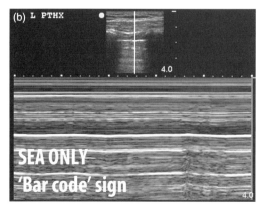

Fig. 26.2. Ultrasound images: (a) B-mode image pneumothorax with line drawing demonstrating the separate structures and reverberation artefact from pneumothorax; (b) M-mode image of pneumothorax demonstrating the *bar code* or *stratosphere sign*.

CT

Features

- Pockets of free gas, represented by collections of low density (~1,000 HU) will form around a collapsed lung (Fig. 27.1).

- Pneumothoraces are most commonly found anteromedially when patients are supine on the CT table.

- Features of underlying lung disease may be present (e.g. emphysema), characterized by well-defined pockets of low density scattered throughout the lung parenchyma, with distorted architecture.

- Pleural effusions may be present, appearing as low-density collections in the dependent portion of the hemithorax. This combination signifies the presence of a hydropneumothorax. If the fluid collection is of increased density, consistent with the presence of blood/haematoma, the combination is then described as a haemopneumothorax.

- Pneumothoraces are most commonly found following iatrogenic or traumatic injuries, and a search for coexistent pathologies is vital to aid definitive management.

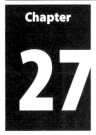

Chapter

27

Pulmonary contusion, rib fractures and flail chest

Characteristics

- Thoracic injury accounts for a significant proportion of all trauma-related deaths.
- Thoracic trauma is divided into blunt or penetrating injuries. In the UK, blunt trauma accounts for the majority of thoracic trauma morbidity/mortality, with road traffic collisions being the largest identifiable factor.
- Injuries can arise either from direct energy transfer to the chest wall and intrathoracic organs, or differential deceleration experienced by intrathoracic organs.
- Commonly described thoracic injury patterns include rib fractures, pulmonary contusions, pneumothoraces and haemothoraces.
  - *Rib fractures* – multiple rib fractures should raise the suspicion of underlying organ injury, e.g. pulmonary contusions, which may not be evident on the initial plain radiograph. Rib fracture sites can help to identify specific visceral organ injuries: upper ribs – major vessel and brachial plexus; lower ribs – spleen, liver and diaphragmatic injury.
  - *Flail segment* – defined as a segment produced by two fractures per rib, with at least two consecutive ribs involved, producing a 'free segment' which can move separately from the chest wall. The significance is that a large segment can disrupt chest wall mechanics enough to require positive pressure ventilation.
  - *Pulmonary contusions* – pathophysiology involves alveolar haemorrhage with interstitial haemorrhage or oedema, resulting in impaired oxygenation secondary to shunting and ventilation of dead space. Can progress to acute respiratory distress syndrome (ARDS) in severe cases.

Clinical features

- Clinical spectrum encompasses a wide variety of presentations.
- Chest wall signs include bruising, significant abrasions, e.g. seatbelt pattern, and paradoxical chest wall movement. Bony crepitus with associated subcutaneous emphysema is suggestive of rib fractures with an underlying pneumothorax.

Radiological features

Ultrasound

Features

- Sensitive for pneumothorax and haemothorax. Areas of lung consolidation may also be easily identifiable.

CT

- Scans should be performed post i.v. contrast in the arterial phase. A pre-contrast study should also be performed if there are concerns regarding an aortic injury.

Features

- **Contusions**
  - Focal or diffuse ground-glass opacities, or consolidation demonstrated by air bronchograms (Fig. 27.1).
  - Air bronchograms may be absent if the bronchus is obstructed, resulting in a wedge-shaped opacity representing collapse.
  - These tend to occur adjacent to vertebrae, ribs, heart and liver.

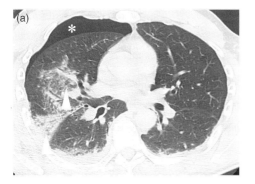

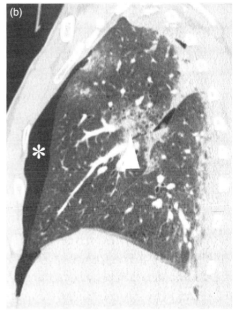

Fig. 27.1. (a) Axial and (b) sagittal images demonstrating areas of ground-glass contusion (arrowheads). Note also the right anterior pneumothorax (asterix) and small right pleural effusion.

- **Rib fractures**
  - o Identified by a breach in the cortex or discontinuity of the ribs.
  - o The degree of displacement should be noted, particularly if there are multiple fractures, as surgical fixation may be considered in order to improve respiratory function.
  - o These are often associated with pneumo/haemothorax.
- **Flail segment**
  - o More than two fractures in two or more consecutive ribs (Fig. 27.2). May involve the sternum or costochondral junctions. Important to recognize as a marker for underlying organ injury.
- **Atelectasis**
  - o Appears as linear bands or wedge-shaped areas of consolidation within the lungs.
  - o Often secondary to inadequate pain relief, limiting ventilatory effort.

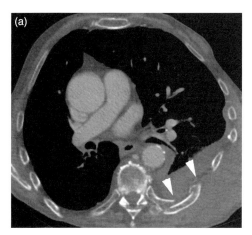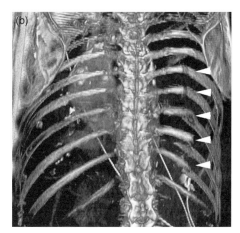

Fig. 27.2. (a) Axial image demonstrating multiple left posterior rib fractures (arrowheads) and a small left pleural effusion. (b) Volume-rendered image of the same patient demonstrating multiple fractures of the left 7th to 11th ribs (arrowheads), in keeping with a flail chest.

Chapter 28 Pulmonary embolism

Characteristics

- Pulmonary embolism (PE) is a blockage in the pulmonary arteries, usually caused by thrombus, but which may be caused by other embolic events such as fat (following major pelvic/lower limb trauma), air or tumour.
- More than 90% of pulmonary emboli originate from the deep veins of the legs.
- If untreated, the mortality rate for a massive PE is 30%, and that for a non-massive PE is <5%.
- Venous thromboembolism is caused by any of the three factors described in the *Virchow triad*:
  - Hypercoagulability
  - Venous stasis or turbulent blood flow
  - Endothelial damage.
- Risk factors for PE include:
  - Surgery – Major abdominal/pelvic surgery; hip/knee replacement
  - Obstetrics – Late pregnancy
  - Reduced mobility – Postoperative, intensive-care, hospitalization
  - Oestrogen – Oral contraceptive pill and hormone replacement therapy
  - Other – Malignancy; previous thromboembolism.
- A D-dimer blood test is a very sensitive but not very specific investigation, and may be raised in many other conditions. A negative D-dimer has a high negative predictive value.

Clinical features

- Shortness of breath, pleuritic chest pain, haemoptysis, calf swelling/tenderness (deep vein thrombosis in the leg).
- In a massive PE: hypoxia, hypotension, tachycardia, collapse and sudden death.

Radiological features

Chest radiograph

Features
- May be normal.
- Pulmonary infarct; segmental, pleurally based wedge-shaped opacity (*Hampton's hump*).
- An area of radiolucency due to focal lung oligaemia (*Westermark's sign*).
- Local widening of the pulmonary artery due to distension from clot (*Fleischner's sign*).

V/Q scan (ventilation/perfusion scan)

Features
- Mismatched perfusion defects
- Performed when the chest radiograph is normal, as other lung pathologies can cause false positive results.

Ultrasound
- Increasingly used in the emergency setting.
- Focused ECHO is used to assess for evidence of raised right ventricular pressure. Look for an abnormal right/left ventricular ratio with interventricular septal bowing towards the left ventricle.
- Poor inferior vena cava collapsibility is suggestive of raised right ventricular pressure.
- Proximal deep venous thrombosis may be demonstrated on extremity ultrasound.

CT pulmonary angiogram (CTPA)
- Contrast-enhanced, thin collimation, spiral CT of the thorax; usually performed with bolus tracking to optimize opacification of the pulmonary arteries (Hounsfield unit >240 HU).

Features
- Filling defects within the pulmonary arterial tree on contrast-enhanced imaging (Fig. 28.1).
- Mosaic perfusion within the lung parenchyma, with reduced vasculature in radiolucent areas.
- 'Bubbly' wedge-shaped peripherally based consolidation, representing lung infarction (Figs. 28.2 and 28.3).
- Increased ratio of main pulmonary artery/ascending aorta diameters, consistent with pulmonary artery hypertension, which is associated with massive PE.

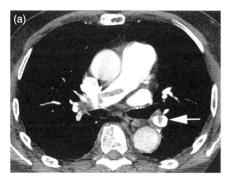
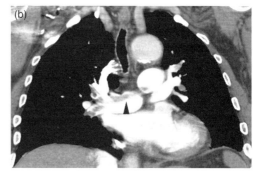

Fig. 28.1. (a) Axial and (b) coronal images demonstrating the presence of filling defects within the main pulmonary artery (arrow and arrowhead) extending to the lobar branches, in keeping with pulmonary embolism.

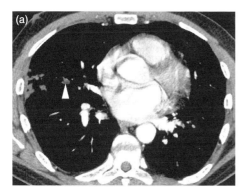
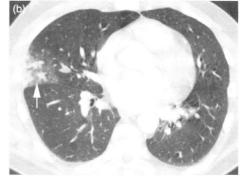

Fig. 28.2. Axial images in (a) mediastinal and (b) lung window settings demonstrating a filling defect in a segmental pulmonary artery (arrowhead) and peripheral wedge-shaped consolidation (arrow).

- Features of right ventricular strain may be present:
  - Increased ratio of right:left ventricle (Fig. 28.4a)
  - Bowing of the interventricular septum towards the left ventricle
  - Reflux of contrast into the inferior vena cava (IVC) and hepatic veins (tricuspid regurgitation) (Fig. 28.4b).

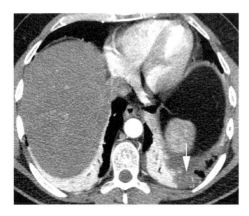

Fig. 28.3. Axial image demonstrating a wedge-shaped area of non-enhancing lung in the posterior segment of the left lower lobe (arrow), lying adjacent to normally enhancing consolidated lung on its medial aspect. There is also consolidation in the right lower lobe.

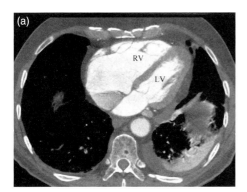

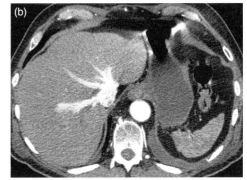

Fig. 28.4. (a) Axial image demonstrating increased right ventricle (RV) to left ventricle (LV) ratio (RV : LV > 1), consistent with right ventricular strain. There is also a small left pleural effusion with adjacent atelectasis. (b) Axial image demonstrating acute tricuspid regurgitation secondary to massive pulmonary embolism. Contrast can be seen refluxing into the inferior vena cava (IVC) and hepatic veins.

Fat emboli

- Much less common than thromboembolic disease.
- Imaging features differ in that there is extensive bilateral air space opacification, similar to acute respiratory distress syndrome (ARDS).

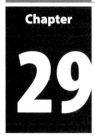

Chapter

29

Abdominal trauma: blunt and penetrating

Characteristics

- Abdominal trauma can be divided into *penetrating* injuries, secondary to stabbings or gunshot wounds, or *blunt* injuries, most commonly caused by motor vehicle collisions.

- Reviews from adult trauma databases reflect that blunt trauma is the leading cause of intra-abdominal injury, accounting for two-thirds of cases. Identification of injuries is often difficult and may not be detected in the initial assessment.

- Abdominal injuries are the leading cause of death in patients aged 1–44 years.

- Peritonitis and haemodynamic instability are associated with hollow viscus perforation and vascular injuries, respectively. Emergent surgical exploration and repair in these patient groups should not necessarily be delayed by CT imaging.

Clinical features

- Evidence of shock: hypotension, tachycardia and narrow pulse pressure, suggests significant intra-abdominal or vascular injury.

- Information provided by personnel attending the scene of the incident is vital, particularly in critically ill patients with altered mental state.

- Type of weapon, entry location, path of injury, extrication, speed of vehicle, and the patient's final position at the scene are examples of information that will help to predict the site and extent of injury.

- External signs of injury, such as abrasions and ecchymoses, help predict the likely injury pattern. The *Cullen sign* – periumbilical ecchymosis, suggests intraperitoneal haemorrhage.

- Lower chest wall deformity, bruising or crepitus suggest lower rib fractures, which can be associated with splenic or hepatic injuries.

  Pelvic instability/fractures are associated with lower urinary tract injuries and retroperitoneal haematoma.

- Focal abdominal tenderness aids localization of the injured organ. In the presence of rigidity and guarding, peritonitis should be suspected secondary to extravasation of intestinal contents or intra-abdominal haemorrhage.

Radiological features

Ultrasound

Features

- FAST (Focused Assessment Sonography in Trauma) has replaced diagnostic peritoneal lavage in many centres as a rapid, non-invasive diagnostic tool.
- Four views – namely pericardial, hepatorenal fossa, splenorenal fossa and pelvic views – are used, and can reliably detect more than 100–250 ml of free fluid. In the context of trauma, this would suggest haemopericardium/peritoneum secondary to visceral organ injury.
- Free fluid appears anechoic and lies in the dependent position in the following locations:
  - ○ Between the echogenic curvilinear diaphragm and the liver or spleen in a subphrenic location (Fig. 29.1a)
  - ○ Between the intermediate echogenic liver/spleen parenchyma and the kidneys in the hepatorenal (Fig. 29.1b)/splenorenal fossae (Fig. 29.1c)
  - ○ Behind the echogenic uterus (pouch of Douglas) (Fig. 29.1d) or anechoic bladder in the pelvis.
- This technique can also detect the presence of a pericardial effusion or pneumothorax, as part of the 'standard' and 'extended' FAST scans, respectively. Please refer to the relevant chapters for details.
- Interval scanning helps to confirm the presence of a haemoperitoneum in cases of doubt. This is necessary in some cases, as a slow rate of bleeding may not initially be detected if the examination is carried out shortly after the injury.
- Difficulties occur in obese patients and in cases of intraperitoneal perforation. Sound wave propagation through subcutaneous fat and air precludes accurate assessment. Small volumes of fluid measuring <3 cm in AP diameter in the pouch of Douglas, in females of reproductive age, may be physiological and should not be assumed to be traumatic free fluid.

CT

- Studies should be performed post intravenous contrast, following a delay of 60–70 s, in the portal venous phase, to ensure homogeneous enhancement of abdominal organs.
- Common findings of abdominal organ trauma will be discussed initially, followed by specific issues in individual organs.

Features

- *Haemoperitoneum* – intraperitoneal free fluid with increased density (30–45 HU) suggests the presence of unclotted blood. Blood and fluid flows into dependent recesses in the abdomen, i.e. subphrenic, perihepatic, perisplenic, paracolic gutters and pelvis.
- *Active haemorrhage* – contrast blush or streaking, originating from opacified vessels on arterial-phase imaging, appears as linear or ill-defined foci of high attenuation.
- *Sentinel clot* – focus of high-attenuation clotted blood (>60 HU) lying adjacent to the injured organ.

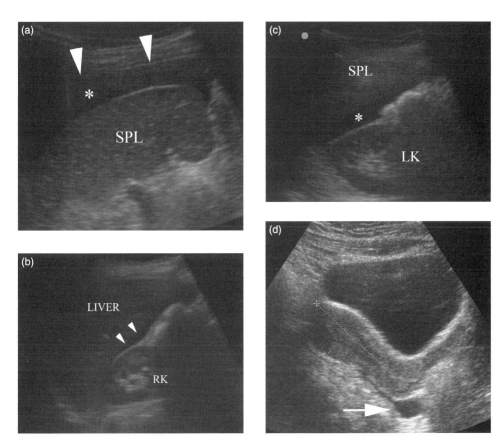

Fig. 29.1. Ultrasound images: (a) left upper quadrant demonstrates an anechoic fluid collection (asterix) lying between the echogenic diaphragm (arrowheads) and the splenic parenchyma (SPL); (b) right upper quadrant shows a small anechoic fluid collection (arrowheads) between the liver and right kidney (RK); (c) anechoic fluid collection (asterix) lying between the spleen (SPL) and left kidney (LK) in the left upper quadrant; (d) anechoic fluid collection in the pelvis in the pouch of Douglas (arrow).

- *Free gas* – suggests perforation of a hollow viscus, secondary to transmural laceration; represented by pockets of low attenuation adjacent to the injured organ. These lie in a non-dependent anterior portion of the abdomen, best seen on lung windows setting.
- *Subcapsular haematoma* – crescentic low-density collection distorting the contour of the neighbouring organ and limited by the external capsule of the organ.
- *Intraparenchymal haematoma/Contusion* – irregular low-density focus within otherwise uniformly enhancing parenchyma.
- *Laceration* – jagged linear low density within otherwise uniformly enhancing parenchyma, which does not necessarily extend from the capsule, but may extend to involve the vascular pedicle (Fig. 29.2).
- *Shattered organ* – multiple lacerations within an organ, with associated intraparenchymal haematoma.

- *Absent parenchymal enhancement and infarction* – global reduction of parenchymal enhancement, suggests laceration/dissection/thrombosis of the supplying artery. When only segmental arteries are involved, this is termed infarction, and appears as wedge-shaped areas of decreased attenuation extending from the capsule.

Spleen

- The most commonly injured abdominal organ; 40% of cases are associated with left lower rib fractures, 25% are associated with left renal injury.
- Delayed rupture may be associated with intraparenchymal or subcapsular haematoma, which can follow a delay of up to 10 days.
- Splenic artery pseudoaneurysm may develop following a vascular injury, leading to further haemorrhage.
- The American Association for the Surgery of Trauma (AAST) splenic injury grading system is shown in Table 29.1.

Table 29.1 AAST grading of splenic injuries.

Grade	Injury
I	• Subcapsular haematoma <10% of surface area • Capsular laceration <1 cm depth
II	• Subcapsular haematoma 10–50% of surface area • Intraparenchymal haematoma <5 cm in diameter • Laceration 1–3 cm depth not involving trabecular vessels
III	• Subcapsular haematoma >50% of surface area or expanding • Intraparenchymal haematoma >5 cm or expanding • Laceration >3 cm depth or involving trabecular vessels • Ruptured subcapsular or parenchymal haematoma
IV	• Laceration involving segmental or hilar vessels with major devascularization (>25% of spleen)
V	• Shattered spleen • Hilar vascular injury with devascularized spleen

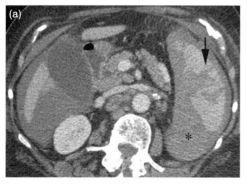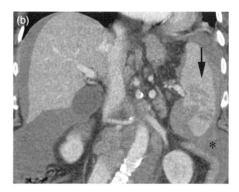

Fig. 29.2. Multiple splenic lacerations: (a) axial and (b) coronal images demonstrating jagged linear areas of low attenuation within an otherwise uniformly enhancing spleen (black arrow). Note the perisplenic and perihepatic low-attenuation free fluid (black asterix).

Liver

- The second most commonly injured abdominal organ, associated with right-sided lower rib fractures; 45% of cases are associated with concurrent splenic injury.

- Right lobe more frequently involved; left lobe associated with duodenal, pancreatic and transverse colon injuries.

- Lacerations tend to parallel the hepatic arteries (Fig. 29.3).

- Periportal low attenuation suggests blood tracking adjacent to the portal vein, injury to the biliary tree or vigorous fluid resuscitation. Careful assessment of biliary duct integrity is vital for prompt management.

- Complications include biloma formation, where bile escapes into a liver haematoma delaying healing, pseudoaneurysm or arterioportal fistula, and infected haematoma.

- CT scan criteria for staging liver trauma based on the AAST liver injury scale are shown in Table 29.2.

Table 29.2 AAST grading of hepatic injuries.

Grade	Injury
I	• Subcapsular haematoma <1 cm in maximal thickness • Capsular avulsion • Superficial parenchymal laceration <1 cm deep • Isolated periportal blood tracking
II	• Parenchymal laceration 1–3 cm deep • Parenchymal/subcapsular haematomas 1–3 cm thick
III	• Parenchymal laceration >3 cm deep • Parenchymal or subcapsular haematoma >3 cm in diameter
IV	• Parenchymal/subcapsular haematoma >10 cm in diameter • Lobar destruction, or devascularization
V	• Global destruction or devascularization of the liver
VI	• Hepatic avulsion

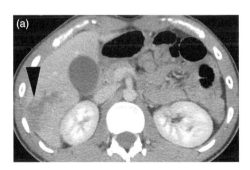
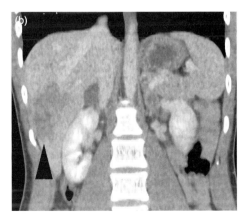

Fig. 29.3. Liver laceration: (a) axial and (b) coronal images demonstrating jagged linear areas of low attenuation within an otherwise uniformly enhancing liver (black arrowhead).

Pancreas

- 75% of cases are associated with penetrating injury, and are often occult.

- The body of the pancreas is most commonly injured, as it is compressed against the spine (Fig. 29.4).

- Fluid tracks along the splenic artery, with thickening of the anterior renal fascia and anterior pararenal space.

- The most important consideration is the integrity of the pancreatic duct, as injury may result in pancreatitis. Other complications include pseudoaneurysm formation, and fistulae.

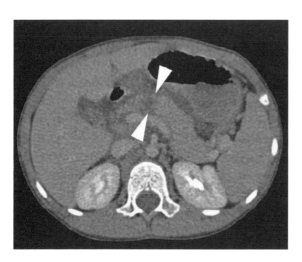

Fig. 29.4. Axial image demonstrating non-enhancement in the pancreatic body (arrowheads), in keeping with a pancreatic laceration.

Bowel and mesentery

- Injury occurs in 5% of blunt trauma cases.

- Free gas or free contrast (if oral contrast has been given) is suggestive of perforation secondary to transmural laceration or complete transection (Fig. 29.5).

- Focal mesenteric haematoma, associated with focal bowel-wall thickening, is suggestive of a significant injury and may require surgical management (Fig. 29.6).

- Retroperitoneal gas and oral contrast are suggestive of a duodenal laceration (especially the third part of the duodenum, which is a common site of injury as it lies anterior to the spine and is prone to compression).

- *Shock bowel* – diffuse small-bowel dilatation, with wall thickening, flattened inferior vena cava, and intense renal enhancement, are specific features of severe hypotension.

- Bowel-wall thickening, in association with periportal oedema, dilated inferior vena cava and normal bowel and renal enhancement, suggests fluid overload resulting from vigorous fluid resuscitation.

- Omental infarction is a rare complication of trauma resulting from venous insufficiency or thrombosis of the omental vein (Fig. 29.7).

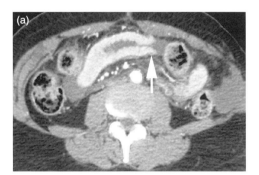
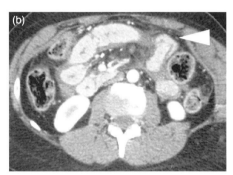

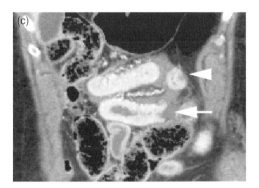

Fig. 29.5. (a), (b) Axial and (c) coronal images demonstrating complete transection of the jejunum with discontinuity of the bowel wall (arrow) and intussusception of the distal transected segment (arrowhead), and surrounding free fluid. There is increased enhancement of the adjacent small-bowel loop, in keeping with oedema.

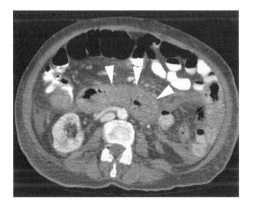

Fig. 29.6. Axial image demonstrating diffuse thickening of the third part of the duodenum (arrowheads) due to post-traumatic duodenal haematoma.

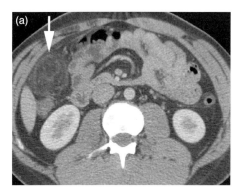 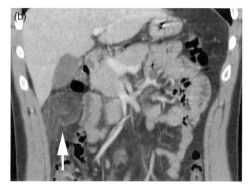

Fig. 29.7. (a) Axial and (b) coronal images demonstrating a well-defined area of increased attenuation in the omentum in the right flank (arrow), consistent with omental infarction. The increased omental attenuation is best appreciated when compared with the density of normal fat surrounding both kidneys.

Renal

- Injury occurs in 8–10% of blunt trauma cases, most commonly minor injuries, presenting with haematuria. Associated with fractures of the 10th to 12th ribs.

- Deceleration injuries can cause vascular pedicle avulsion or thrombosis. This can occur secondary to a dissection, resulting in absent renal enhancement and a large perinephric haematoma. Significant mortality is associated with vascular pedicle injury and careful assessment for renal arterial enhancement is therefore important in suspected cases.

- Deep lacerations may extend to involve the collecting system, best demonstrated on delayed-phase imaging, with contrast leaking into the perirenal space.

- Pelvi-ureteric junction tears can result from deceleration injuries, causing contrast leakage around the renal pelvis or kidney, with absence of contrast in the distal ureter on delayed-phase imaging.

- Renal injuries are graded by the AAST on the basis of the depth of injury, and the involvement of vessels or the collecting system, as shown in Table 29.3.

Table 29.3 AAST grading of renal injuries.

Grade	Injury
I	• Haematuria with normal imaging studies • Contusions • Nonexpanding subcapsular haematomas
II	• Nonexpanding perinephric haematomas confined to the retroperitoneum • Superficial cortical lacerations <1 cm in depth without collecting system injury
III	• Renal lacerations >1 cm in depth that do not involve the collecting system (Figs. 29.8 and 29.9)
IV	• Renal lacerations extending through the kidney into the collecting system • Injuries involving the main renal artery or vein with contained haemorrhage • Segmental infarctions without associated lacerations • Expanding subcapsular haematomas compressing the kidney
V	• Shattered or devascularized kidney (Fig. 29.10) • Ureteropelvic avulsions • Complete laceration or thrombus of the main renal artery or vein

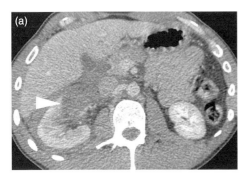
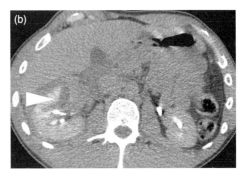

Fig. 29.8. Renal laceration: (a) portal venous phase and (b) delayed-phase axial images demonstrating a low-attenuation region in the anterior interpolar region of the right kidney consistent with renal laceration (arrowhead). There is an associated perinephric haematoma. Note that the contrast is confined to the collection system and does not leak into the perinephric space on the delayed-phase image, excluding laceration extension into the collection system.

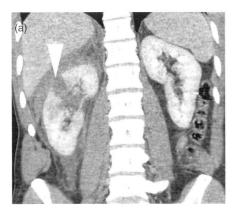
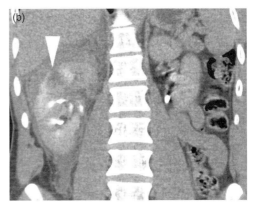

Fig. 29.9. Renal laceration: (a) portal venous phase and (b) delayed-phase coronal images demonstrating a right interpolar region renal laceration (arrowhead) with perinephric haematoma. Note that there is no leakage of contrast into the perinephric space on the delayed-phase images.

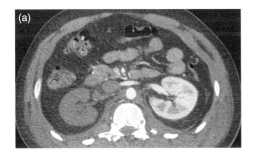
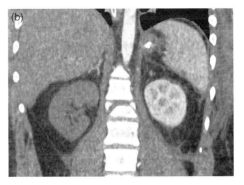

Fig. 29.10. Grade V renal injury: (a) axial and (b) coronal images in portal venous phase demonstrating complete lack of right renal parenchyma enhancement, consistent with a devascularized kidney. This is secondary to traumatic dissection of the right renal artery.

Bladder

- *Intraperitoneal rupture* arises as a result of a direct blow to a distended bladder. The resulting increased intravesical pressure causes a horizontal tear along the intraperitoneal portion of the bladder wall. Most common in intoxicated patients or those sustaining blunt trauma following a road traffic accident. On delayed-phase imaging, contrast is seen around bowel loops and dependent intraperitoneal areas.

- *Extraperitoneal rupture* – usually associated with pelvic fractures in up to 90% of patients. Conversely, approximately 10% of patients with pelvic fractures also have significant bladder injuries. Results from the shearing force of the deforming bony pelvic ring, causing a 'burst' injury. On delayed-phase imaging, contrast leaks into the perivesical space (Fig. 29.11), abdominal wall, scrotum and thigh, and can track superiorly within the retroperitoneum.

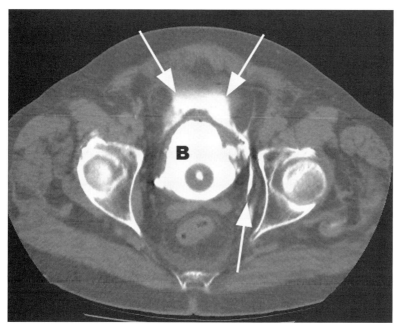

Fig. 29.11. CT cystogram image demonstrating extravasation of contrast into the perivesical space (arrows) secondary to extraperitoneal bladder perforation following transurethral resection of a bladder tumour. A Foley catheter is in situ and there are multiple bilateral bladder diverticula.

Adrenal

- Injury occurs in 2% of severe trauma cases.
- There is a preponderance for the right adrenal gland.
- Acute haemorrhage appears as high density (>50 HU) replacing the gland, or streaky high density in the periadrenal fat (Fig. 29.12).

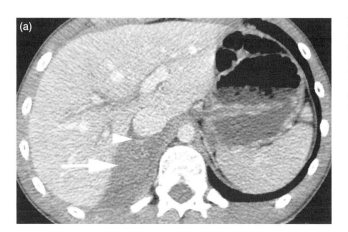

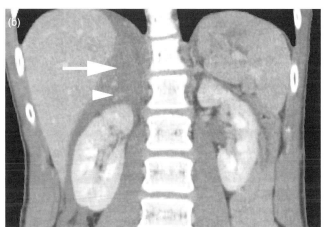

Fig. 29.12. (a) Axial and (b) coronal images demonstrating a small area of enhancing adrenal gland (arrowhead), with fluid attenuation in the right adrenal bed (arrow), consistent with a right adrenal haematoma and surrounding haemorrhage.

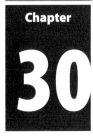

Abdominal aortic aneurysm

Characteristics

- An aneurysm is defined as dilatation of the aorta >150% of its normal diameter. The normal diameter of the infrarenal aorta is 1.5 cm in females and 1.7 cm in males. An infrarenal aorta measuring >3 cm in diameter is considered to be an abdominal aortic aneurysm (AAA), even if asymptomatic.

- The incidence is 2–4% in the adult population, most commonly detected incidentally due to the increasing use of imaging. AAA affects males more frequently, with an incidence ratio of 2:1 in those <80 years of age, rising to an equal sex incidence in the population >80 years of age.

- Reported incidence of rupture varies between 1 and 21 per 100,000 population. Rupture of an AAA is a devastating event, with 65% mortality from cardiovascular collapse prior to reaching hospital.

- Atherosclerosis is the commonest described causative factor, accounting for 90% of cases.

- Family history is also a significant risk factor, with increased risk proportional to the number of first-degree relatives affected. The familial prevalence rate is 15–25%.

- Other risk factors include: smoking, chronic obstructive pulmonary disease (COPD), hypertension, infection, cystic medial necrosis, arteritis, trauma and connective tissue disorders (Marfan and Ehlers–Danlos syndromes).

- AAA has been shown to result from medial degeneration of the arterial wall, responsible for the structural and elastic properties of arteries. Progressive degeneration results in progressive dilatation of the aorta

- Infection accounts for 5% of AAAs. Local invasion of the intima and media gives rise to abscess formation and aneurysmal dilatation.

- AAAs are typically fusiform in morphology with circumferential dilatation of the vessel wall. Saccular aneurysms, with localized outpouchings, are seen less frequently but carry an increased risk of rupture.

Clinical features

- Most patients with AAA are asymptomatic, and diagnosed incidentally. Progressive symptoms (abdominal and back pain, vomiting, syncope and claudication) are common, suggesting expansion and possible rupture.

- An expanding aneurysm can cause severe low back, abdominal, flank or groin pain.
- A ruptured AAA often presents with shock, manifesting clinically as tachycardia, hypotension, cyanosis and altered mental state.
- A pulsatile abdominal mass is found in only 30–50% of patients, and is more commonly seen in ruptured AAA.
- Peripheral emboli to the lower limb may produce *blue toe syndrome*.
- Rarely, aortocaval fistulation occurs which can present as congestive cardiac failure, renal failure or peripheral ischaemia. An abdominal bruit found on clinical examination is suggestive of this. The aorta may also rupture into the fourth part of the duodenum, resulting in catastrophic gastrointestinal haemorrhage.

Radiological features

Ultrasound

Features

- Excellent tool to identify and measure the size of an aortic aneurysm.
- Increasingly used as the gold standard in the emergency presentation of a suspected ruptured AAA.
- Care must be exercised in the identification of the aorta, to avoid measurement of other rounded structures such as a vertebral body (Fig. 30.1). Measurement should be from outer wall to outer wall to avoid erroneously measuring the lumen only (Fig. 30.2).
- Rupture is not reliably detected on ultrasound and diagnosis should be based on ultrasound findings combined with clinical history and examination.

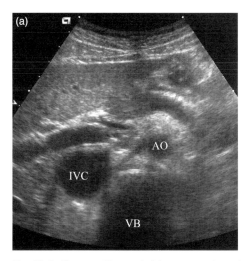
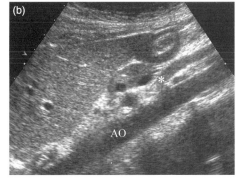

Fig. 30.1. Ultrasound images in (a) transverse plane, demonstrating other rounded structures (inferior vena cava (IVC), vertebral body (VB)) which can be mistaken for the aorta (AO) and measured erroneously. (b) Longitudinal image of the aorta, demonstrating the anterior origin of the superior mesenteric artery (asterix).

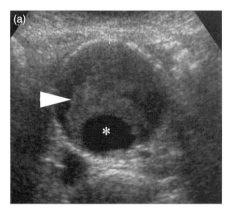 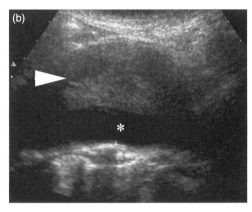

Fig. 30.2. Ultrasound images in (a) transverse plane and (b) longitudinal plane, demonstrating the aneurysm sac of the abdominal aorta (cross markers) surrounding the anechoic aortic lumen (asterix). Note the intraluminal echogenic material in keeping with thrombus within the aneurysm sac (arrowhead).

CT

- A pre-contrast study followed by CT angiography should be performed.
- The study should be reviewed in axial plane with multiplanar reformats and maximum-intensity projections.

Features

- Aneurysmal dilatation of the aorta can be readily assessed. A low-density crescentic mural thrombus is often seen within the aneurysm sac (Fig. 30.3).
- Crescentic high density within the sac, but outside the lumen, is a sign of imminent rupture (Fig. 30.4).
- Discontinuity of the aortic wall suggests frank rupture associated with contrast extravasation, or haematoma within the para-aortic region, retroperitoneum and dependent areas of the abdomen and pelvis (Fig. 30.5).
- Small leaks may only present with high-density stranding within the periaortic fat, or high-density intra-abdominal fluid, consistent with haemoperitoneum.
- High-density material or contrast within the bowel lumen suggests an aortoenteric fistula.
- High-density contrast within the inferior vena cava in the early arterial-phase study is suspicious of an aortocaval fistula.
- Gas locules within the aneurysm sac are suggestive of an infective aetiology, often precluding endovascular management.
- Additional information required to guide either endovascular or open surgical repair includes:
  - Relationship of the renal arteries to the aneurysm sac
  - Shape and length of aneurysm neck
  - Number of renal arteries
  - Presence of a retroaortic left renal vein

- ○ Iliac artery involvement
- ○ Calibre and degree of atherosclerosis within the external iliac arteries for endovascular access.
- The planning of endovascular repair is beyond the scope of this chapter, but early referral to both vascular surgeons and interventional radiologists is vital for optimal management.

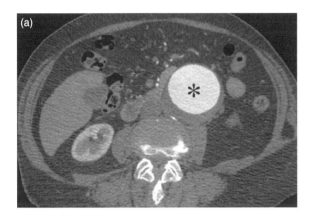

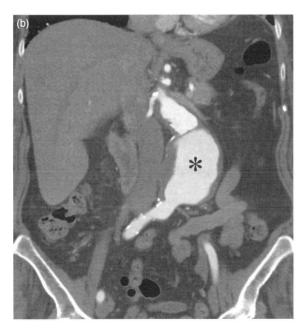

Fig. 30.3. (a) Axial and (b) coronal arterial-phase images demonstrating an aneurysmal abdominal aorta (black asterix) with crescentic low-attenuation thrombus adherent to its posterior wall.

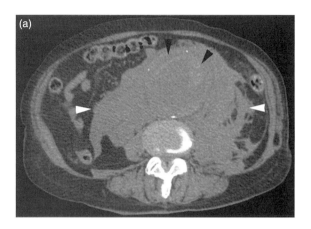

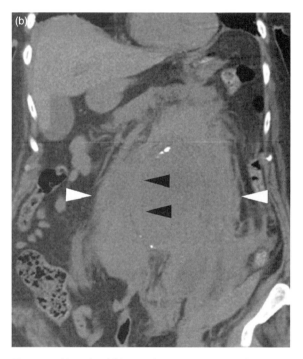

Fig. 30.4. (a) Axial and (b) coronal pre-contrast images demonstrating crescentic high attenuation within the aneurysmal sac, suggesting rupture (black arrowheads). There is a large para-aortic high-attenuation collection extending into the retroperitoneum in keeping with haematoma (white arrowheads).

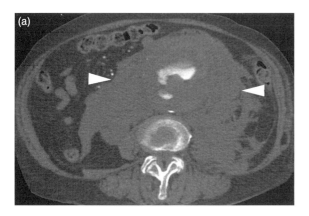

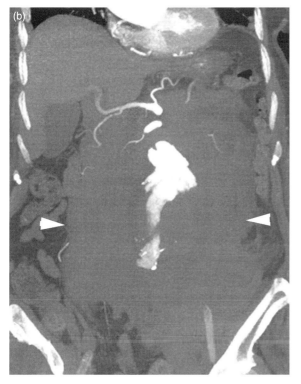

Fig. 30.5. (a) Axial and (b) coronal arterial-phase images demonstrating a large para-aortic high-attenuation haematoma (arrowheads) surrounding the aneurysmal abdominal aorta, which contains intraluminal contrast.

Chapter

31

Appendicitis

Characteristics

- Common cause of an acute abdomen, with peak incidence in the second and third decades of life.
- Inflammation of the appendix is usually caused by luminal obstruction, secondary to lymphoid hyperplasia or a faecolith.
- Complications include localized perforation, abscess formation and generalized peritonitis.

Clinical features

- Classical presentation is with central colicky abdominal pain which migrates to the right iliac fossa (RIF), associated with nausea, vomiting, fever and raised inflammatory markers.
- Only 50% present in a typical fashion, with a significant proportion presenting with non-specific symptoms. The differential diagnosis is therefore vast, including cholecystitis, Crohn's colitis, urinary tract infection, ovarian torsion and pelvic inflammatory disease, to name but a few. This often makes the diagnosis difficult, resulting in a greater dependence on imaging to confirm the findings.

Radiological features

Ultrasound

- Imaging modality of choice if there is diagnostic uncertainty, particularly in children and young slim adults.
- The entire abdomen should be scanned to exclude other differential diagnoses.

Features

- Visualization of a blind-ending, non-peristaltic, non-compressible, tubular structure, usually in the RIF or right upper quadrant (RUQ) (Fig. 31.1).
- Tubular diameter of ≥6 mm.
- Presence of an appendicolith.

- Echogenic mesentery surrounding the appendix, in keeping with an inflammatory response, and separation of adjacent bowel loops.
- Increased Doppler flow within the mesentery and in the wall of the tubular structure suggestive of inflammation.
- Pelvic free fluid or focal collection.

N.B. A negative ultrasound scan does not exclude appendicitis. If there is a high degree of clinical suspicion, this should not preclude further imaging/laparoscopy.

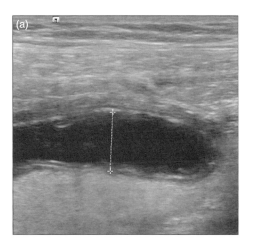

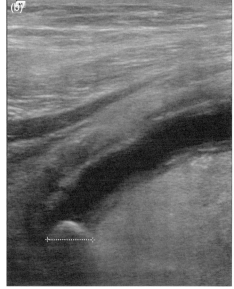

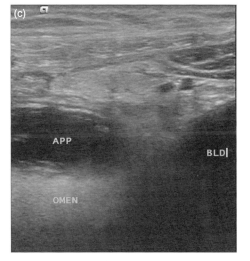

Fig. 31.1. Ultrasound images showing (a) an anechoic blind-ending tubular structure measuring 10 mm in diameter in the right iliac fossa (RIF): this was found to be non-peristaltic and non-compressible; (b) an echogenic round body, with posterior acoustic shadowing, seen within the tubular structure, in keeping with an appendicolith; (c) APP = dilated appendix, OMEN = surrounding echogenic inflamed omentum, BLD = bladder.

CT

Features (Fig. 31.2)

- Dilated (≥10 mm), usually fluid-filled, blind-ending, tubular structure originating from the caecal pole.
- Inflammatory stranding in the peri-appendiceal fat.
- Surrounding free fluid or a focal enhancing collection.
- Presence of an appendicolith.
- Locules of free gas adjacent to the appendix, which confirms perforation.

If the appendix is visualized and appears normal, the rest of the abdomen should be closely scrutinized to exclude other differential diagnoses.

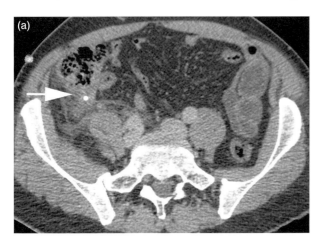

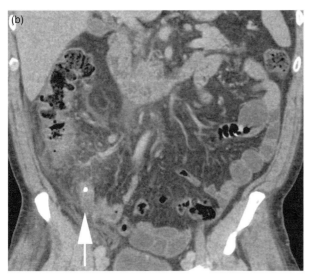

Fig. 31.2. CT images: (a) axial and (b) coronal images demonstrating a fluid-filled dilated appendix containing a well-defined high-attenuation body, in keeping with an appendicolith (arrow). Surrounding peri-appendiceal inflammatory soft-tissue stranding is evident.

Chapter 32

Biliary obstruction/acute cholecystitis

Characteristics

- Inflammation of the gallbladder occurs secondary to obstruction by gallstones, either at the gallbladder neck or the cystic duct.

- Classical risk factors for gallstones include Caucasian origin, female, women of childbearing age, obesity and age >40 years. However the majority of patients with gallstones are usually asymptomatic, with only 1–3% of individuals developing intermittent abdominal pain known as biliary colic. Of these, 20% will progress to acute cholecystitis if untreated.

- Acalculous cholecystitis is a form of gallbladder inflammation in the absence of gallstones, classically described in critically ill patients. Increased incidence is also recorded in children and diabetic patients.

- Complications include empyema, perforation, pericholecystic abscess and cholecystoenteric fistula.

Clinical features

- Patients typically present with prolonged epigastric or RUQ pain radiating to the right shoulder, with associated nausea, vomiting, pyrexia and raised inflammatory markers.

Radiological features

Ultrasound

- The mainstay of imaging in cholecystitis.

Features

- Gallbladder wall thickening (>3 mm), which may be poorly defined.

- Impacted calculi in the gallbladder neck or cystic duct. Gallstones are visualized as echogenic foci with posterior acoustic shadowing (Fig. 32.1a).

- Biliary sludge may be seen as echogenic debris layering in the gallbladder. This is particulate matter precipitated in bile prior to stone formation.

- Pericholecystic fluid.

- Positive ultrasound *Murphy's sign* – focal tenderness and inspiratory arrest upon direct pressure with the ultrasound probe in the RUQ, which is not elicited with pressure in the left upper quadrant (LUQ) – is present in 85% of cases.
- Calculi can migrate into the common bile duct (CBD), causing obstruction. The intrahepatic ducts and the CBD will be dilated (Fig. 32.1b). The CBD is considered dilated if >6 mm in diameter (up to age 60 with an allowance of an additional 1 mm with each decade after this). An intraductal calculus demonstrates similar features to gallstones within the gallbladder.

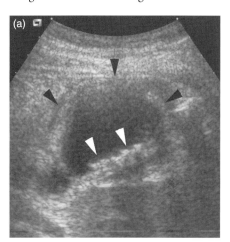 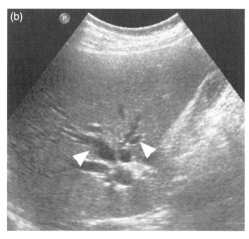

Fig. 32.1. (a) Ultrasound image demonstrating a thick-walled gallbladder (black arrowheads), consistent with acute cholecystitis. This contains multiple echogenic foci (white arrowheads) with posterior acoustic shadowing, in keeping with gallstones. Note also the presence of small-volume pericholecystic anechoic fluid. (b) Ultrasound image of the liver hilum demonstrating dilated intrahepatic ducts (arrowheads).

CT

- This is not routinely required, but may be utilized as part of the investigation of non-specific abdominal pain, or to assess for secondary complications of cholecystitis.

Features

- Gallbladder wall thickening (>3 mm).
- Biliary calculi may be visualized as foci of high attenuation within the gallbladder, although this is best visualized with ultrasound.
- Inflammatory stranding in the pericholecystic fat (Fig. 32.2).
- Pericholecystic fluid/focal enhancing collections will appear as a low-attenuation collection surrounding the gallbladder.
- Locules of free gas adjacent to the gallbladder secondary to necrosis/perforation.
- Cholecystoenteric fistulae are rare. Inflammatory adhesions form between the gallbladder and adjacent small-bowel wall, enabling a calculus to erode through the gallbladder wall into the bowel lumen. This in turn can lead to a rare cause of small-bowel obstruction secondary to calculus impaction, classically in the terminal ileum rather than the ileocaecal valve. Review images for air within the biliary tree secondary to fistulation (Fig. 32.3).

- Migration of a calculus into the common bile duct (CBD) will result in biliary obstruction with dilatation of the intrahepatic ducts and CBD. The calculus can occasionally be visualized with CT (Fig. 32.4) although MRCP (magnetic resonance cholangiopancreatography) is generally performed to investigate this.

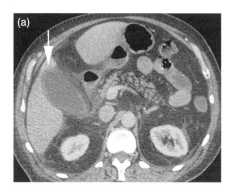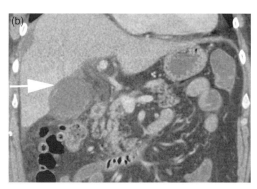

Fig 32.2. (a) Axial and (b) coronal images showing a thick-walled distended gallbladder with pericholecystic stranding, in keeping with acute cholecystitis (arrow).

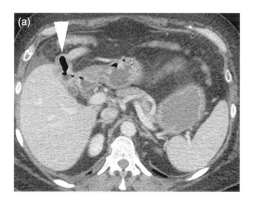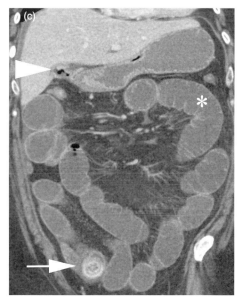

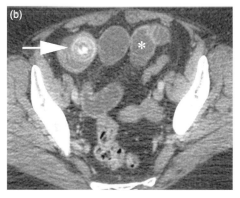

Fig. 32.3. (a), (b) Axial and (c) coronal images demonstrating gas locules within a collapsed gallbladder, in keeping with cholecystoenteric fistulation (arrowhead). A lamellated gallstone is seen within the distal small bowel (arrow), with dilatation of small-bowel loops (asterix), in keeping with gallstone ileus.

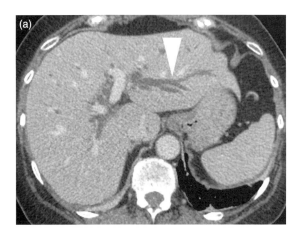

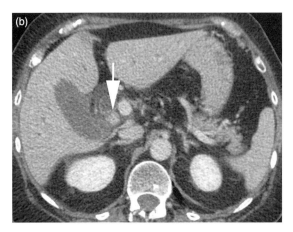

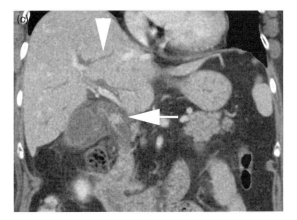

Fig 32.4. (a), (b) Axial and (c) coronal images showing dilatation of the intrahepatic ducts (arrowhead) and CBD, where a gallstone is identified (arrow).

Chapter

33

Bowel obstruction

- Small- and large-bowel obstruction (SBO and LBO) often share the similar clinical features of abdominal distension, colicky pain, vomiting and constipation. As their aetiology and management are usually quite different, they will be considered separately.

Small-bowel obstruction

Characteristics

- Small-bowel obstruction (SBO) presents with abdominal distension, bilious vomiting and colicky abdominal pain. The higher the level of obstruction, the more rapid the onset of vomiting, with less severe abdominal distension. In distal SBO obstruction, there is greater distension and colicky abdominal pain, with vomiting as a late feature.
- The bowel distal to the obstruction empties and collapses while the bowel proximal to the obstruction distends with gas and fluid.
- 'Fluid shift' into the bowel can cause hypovolaemia, tachycardia and electrolyte imbalances.
- The mechanical causes of SBO can be divided into intraluminal, mural and extraluminal causes, as shown in Table 33.1.
- The commonest cause of SBO is adhesions, followed by hernias.

Radiological features

CT

- CT can confirm the diagnosis of SBO, indicate the location of the obstruction and may identify a cause.
- Scans are normally performed following intravenous contrast alone. Oral contrast is not usually tolerated or required, as dilated bowel loops are filled with fluid, which acts as inherent negative contrast.
- A small-bowel diameter >2.5 cm on CT is abnormal.
- A focal calibre change from dilated to collapsed bowel, the *transition point*, indicates the level of obstruction.

Table 33.1 The mechanical causes of small-bowel obstruction.

Intraluminal	Mural	Extramural
Foreign body	Tumour	Adhesions
Bezoar	Inflammatory stricture (e.g. Crohn's disease)	Hernias
Food bolus	Haematoma	Malrotation/mid-gut volvulus
Gallstone	Intussusception	Congenital bands

- The *small-bowel faeces sign* describes particulate matter found in the lumen of the dilated small bowel and is usually present at the transition point.
- Adhesive bands are not visible on CT; however, there may be kinking of the bowel or angulation, suggesting the presence of a band. The diagnosis is inferred on the basis of a transition point when no other cause is demonstrated (Fig. 33.1).
- A review of hernial orifices may reveal an incarcerated or strangulated hernia (Fig. 33.2).
- Irregular bowel-wall thickening and lymphadenopathy is suggestive of tumour.
- A *bowel-within-bowel* appearance (*doughnut or target sign*), usually containing mesenteric fat and vessels, is pathognomonic for intussusception (see Chapter 39: Intussusception).
- Transmural bowel-wall thickening with stricture or fistula formation suggests Crohn's disease.
- Inflammatory stranding may be seen in the mesenteric fat and non-specific free fluid within the abdomen and pelvis.
- Diffuse small-bowel dilatation, without collapse of the large bowel, is usually due to a functional ileus rather than mechanical obstruction.
- In closed-loop obstruction, a U-shaped loop of bowel is seen with a transition point at either end. There is twisting of the mesentery and contained vessels towards the site of obstruction.
- In strangulated bowel obstruction, there may be circumferential bowel-wall thickening due to venous congestion and resulting oedema. This progresses to bowel ischaemia and necrosis. There may be reduced or asymmetric bowel-wall enhancement, and high-attenuation fluid or haemorrhage within the mesentery. In severe cases, gas may be seen within the bowel wall and within the portal venous system (see Chapter 34: Mesenteric ischaemia).
- The presence of gas in the biliary tree, associated with dilated small-bowel loops, is suggestive of cholecystoenteric fistula. This can cause a gallstone ileus – a rare cause of small-bowel obstruction (Fig. 32.3).

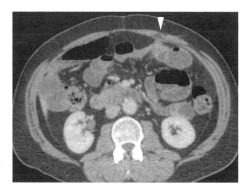

Fig. 33.1. Axial image demonstrating an abrupt transition point within the small bowel. There is angulation of the bowel towards the anterior abdominal wall (arrowhead) at the site of previous surgery. Appearance is in keeping with small-bowel obstruction secondary to adhesions.

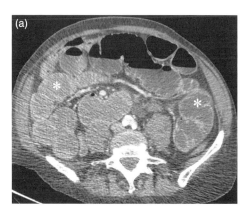

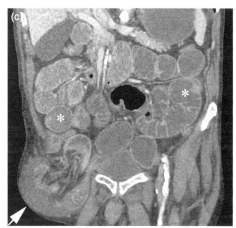

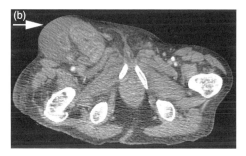

Fig. 33.2. (a), (b) Axial and (c) coronal images showing multiple dilated loops of small bowel (asterix), secondary to a right inguinal hernia (arrow).

Large-bowel obstruction

Characteristics

- Abdominal distension predominates, with colicky abdominal pain and absolute constipation – a feature of complete obstruction.
- Faeculent vomiting occurs if the ileocaecal valve is incompetent, whereby features of SBO are added to those of LBO.

- The most common causes of mechanical LBO are carcinoma of the colon, diverticulitis and volvulus.
- The clinical history is often key to identifying the underlying cause. An abrupt onset of symptoms suggests an acute event such as volvulus, whereas a more prolonged history, with a change in bowel habit and weight loss, is more in keeping with colonic carcinoma.
- Right-sided colonic lesions classically present late and can become quite large before obstruction develops. Sigmoid and rectal tumours tend to obstruct earlier because of the narrower colonic calibre and more solid stool.

Radiological features

CT

- Performed following intravenous contrast. Depending on the clinical scenario, oral contrast may be helpful in outlining small-bowel loops.
- CT confirms obstruction, with a colonic diameter of >6 cm (9 cm in the caecum) considered abnormal.
- Identification of a transition point indicates the level of obstruction.
- CT can also assess for the presence of complications, such as strangulation (see SBO), intramural gas, perforation and abscess formation.

Features
Colonic carcinoma
- Focal irregular bowel-wall thickening with proximal dilatation (Fig. 33.3).
- There may be inflammatory stranding in the adjacent fat.
- Assess for lymphadenopathy and distant metastases.

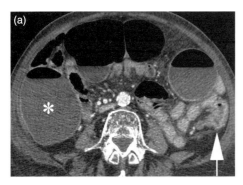

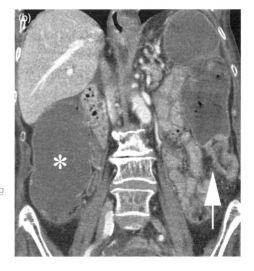

Fig. 33.3 (a) Axial and (b) coronal images demonstrating large-bowel obstruction (asterix) secondary to a colonic carcinoma in the distal descending colon (arrow).

Diverticulitis

- Recurrent diverticulitis can lead to chronic strictures, which can cause large-bowel obstruction (see Chapter 36: Diverticulitis).

Volvulus

- Volvulus accounts for 10% of large-bowel obstructions.
- The sigmoid and caecum are the most common sites for volvulus.
- Volvulus occurs where a section of the large bowel has a mesenteric attachment, providing an opportunity for the bowel to twist on its mesenteric axis.
- Elderly patients with neuropsychiatric disorders, or those who are institutionalized, are more at risk of volvulus.

Sigmoid volvulus

- Accounts for 75% of large-bowel volvulus cases.
- Most cases are diagnosed on plain radiographs with specific features:
  - A dilated coffee-bean-shaped viscus originating in the left iliac fossa and extending into the right upper quadrant.
  - The *left flank overlay sign* (dilated descending colon).
  - The caecum is seen as a separate structure, thus distinguishing this from caecal volvulus.

Caecal volvulus

- Less common than sigmoid volvulus with characteristic plain radiograph features including:
  - A dilated viscus originating in the right iliac fossa and extending towards the left upper quadrant.
  - Small-bowel dilatation.
  - Collapse of the left side of the colon.
- Occasionally, when the diagnosis is not certain, CT can be performed. A grossly dilated viscus (sigmoid colon or caecum) is seen, with twisting of the adjacent mesentery and vessels, giving a 'whorled' appearance (Figs. 33.4 and 33.5).

Pseudo-obstruction

- Occurs in elderly patients with systemic medical conditions and is thought to be due to autonomic imbalance.
- Symptoms, signs and radiographic appearance of LBO but with no identifiable mechanical cause.

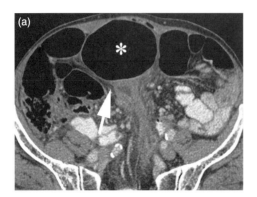
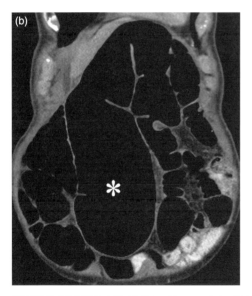
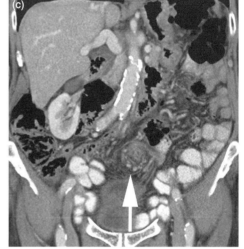

Fig. 33.4. (a) Axial and (b), (c) coronal images demonstrating a dilated sigmoid colon (asterix) with a transition point at the recto-sigmoid junction (arrow). This corresponds to the site of the whirling appearance seen on the coronal image (arrow). Appearance is in keeping with a sigmoid volvulus.

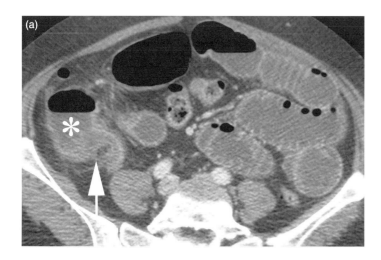

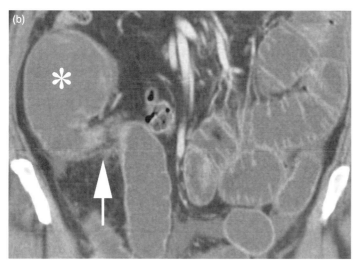

Fig. 33.5. (a) Axial and (b) coronal images showing dilated caecum (asterix) with an acute transition point and whirling of the adjacent mesentery (arrow) consistent with a caecal volvulus.

Chapter 34

Mesenteric ischaemia

Characteristics

- Decreased blood supply to the small or large bowel, resulting in ischaemia and infarction.
- Usually occurs in either the superior mesenteric (SMA) or inferior mesenteric (IMA) arterial distributions, or both.
- The most common site of disease is the watershed area between the two, involving the splenic flexure, due to its poor arterial supply.
- Causes include:
  1. Low flow states (50%)
     - Non-occlusive disease/vasospasm.
     - Patients often have atherosclerotic mesenteric vessels.
     - Reduced perfusion can occur secondary to congestive cardiac failure or hypovolaemia.
     - Peripheral vasodilatation results in shunting of blood from GI tract.
     - Digitalis has been found to cause vasoconstriction of arterial and venous smooth muscle.
  2. Arterial occlusion (40%)
     - Thromboembolic disease.
     - Thrombus usually occurs at the origin of the SMA.
     - Emboli usually lodge in the SMA, distal to the origin of the middle colic artery.
     - Emboli occur secondary to atrial fibrillation or mural thrombus from myocardial infarction.
  3. Venous thrombosis (10%)

Clinical features

- Present acutely with severe abdominal pain, hypotension and acidosis.
- Chronic ischaemia may present with postprandial abdominal pain, resulting in a fear of eating and resultant weight loss.

Radiological features

CT

- CT angiography allows the assessment of splanchnic vessels, namely the coeliac axis, superior and inferior mesenteric arteries.
- This should be followed by a portal venous phase study to assess bowel-wall enhancement and venous thrombosis.

Features

- Low-density filling defects within an enhancing artery confirms the presence of thrombus. Reduced or non-enhancement suggests thrombosis or atherosclerotic narrowing.
- The affected colon demonstrates symmetrical circumferential thickening, with enlarged folds.
- The bowel wall may demonstrate either low attenuation due to oedema, or high attenuation due to mural haemorrhage.
- Bowel-wall enhancement may be poor, with a sharp cut-off between normal and abnormal colon at the boundary of vascular territories.
- In severe cases, gas may be seen within the bowel wall, appearing as intramural locules of low attenuation, in keeping with necrosis (Fig. 34.1). Gas may also be seen in the portal venous system, as branching peripheral low attenuation, usually in the left lobe of the liver (Fig. 34.2). This is a poor prognostic factor.

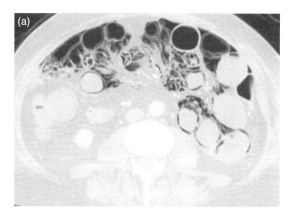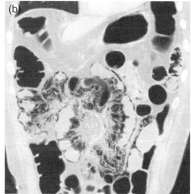

Fig. 34.1. (a) Axial and (b) coronal images on lung windows demonstrating diffuse intramural low attenuation within the small bowel (pneumatosis intestinalis), in keeping with necrosis secondary to mesenteric ischaemia.

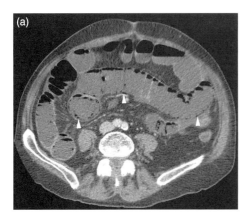

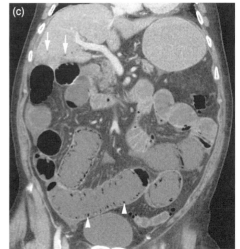

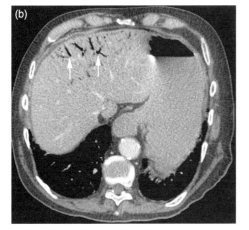

Fig. 34.2. (a), (b) Axial and (c) coronal images demonstrating gas within the bowel wall (arrowheads) and portal venous system (arrows) consistent with ischaemic small bowel.

Pathology – Abdomen and pelvis

Chapter 35

Colitis

Characteristics

- A group of conditions linked by inflammation of the colon. These include inflammatory bowel disease (namely ulcerative colitis and Crohn's disease), ischaemia and infection.

Inflammatory bowel disease

- Idiopathic chronic inflammatory disorder of the bowel.
- Encompasses both ulcerative colitis and Crohn's disease.

Ulcerative colitis

- Inflammation and diffuse ulceration of the colonic mucosa. The rectum is involved in 95% of untreated patients, with contiguous proximal colonic ulceration. Although classically limited to the colon, backwash ileitis describes the phenomenon where the terminal ileum is affected, whilst the remainder of the small bowel is normal. Rectal sparing may be seen in patients treated with steroid enemas.
- Incidence of 10.4–12 cases per 100,000 people; affecting 30% more females than males.
- Extracolonic manifestations are common, with ankylosing spondylitis, erythema nodosum, pyoderma gangrenosum and primary sclerosing cholangitis.
- Complications include toxic megacolon, associated with a high risk of perforation and death. Strictures may form in chronic cases.
- The risk of colorectal cancer increases by 0.5–1% per year, requiring annual colonoscopic surveillance, which should begin 8–10 years after the onset of symptoms.

Crohn's disease

- Transmural inflammation affecting any part of the gastrointestinal tract from the mouth to the anus.
- Most commonly involves the small bowel, especially the terminal ileum, with skip lesions. Colonic disease tends to involve the right colon.
- Incidence ranges from 0.7 to 9.8 cases per 100,000 persons, with a preponderance in females; female to male ratio is 1.2:1.
- The most common extra-intestinal manifestation is inflammatory arthropathy, including ankylosing spondylitis, psoriatic arthritis, reactive arthritis and sacroiliitis. Other

manifestations include ocular manifestations (episcleritis, uveitis, iritis), skin manifestations (erythema nodosum, pyoderma gangrenosum), nephrolithiasis, sclerosing cholangitis, autoimmune chronic hepatitis and cholelithiasis.

- Complications include malabsorption, fistulation, obstruction and inflammatory adhesions.

Clinical features

- Left iliac fossa pain and bloody diarrhoea, with or without mucus, is the most common presentation in ulcerative colitis. Cramping right iliac fossa pain and non-bloody diarrhoea are more common in Crohn's disease.
- Weight loss and fatigue may be associated features. The history may suggest periods of disease activity interspersed with periods of remission.
- Symptoms of obstruction may be seen in Crohn's disease due to inflammatory oedema. Other findings include perianal fissures and fistulae.
- Electrolyte imbalance, specifically hypokalaemia and hypomagnesaemia, may be seen in both conditions, due to severe diarrhoea.
- A definitive diagnosis of ulcerative colitis is made with endoscopy and histology. Imaging plays a role in acute flare-ups in identifying complications, although the diagnosis may be made when imaging is performed for other clinical indications.

Radiological features

CT

Features

- There is extensive overlap between ulcerative colitis and Crohn's disease. Ulcerative colitis more typically affects the left colon, with no small-bowel involvement, as opposed to right colonic and small-bowel involvement (Fig. 35.3), with skip lesions, in Crohn's disease.
- Wall thickening is usually greater in Crohn's disease (11–13 mm) than ulcerative colitis (7–8 mm). The pattern is more typically eccentric and segmental in Crohn's disease, with circumferential, symmetrical and diffuse involvement in ulcerative colitis (Fig. 35.1).
- The *halo sign* – a low-attenuation ring in the submucosal layer, secondary to fat deposition, is more commonly seen in ulcerative colitis.
- Pericolic fat proliferation is seen in Crohn's disease – exuberant fat (low density) is deposited around inflamed bowel loops, resulting in bowel loop separation.
- Mesenteric lymph nodes are more commonly associated with Crohn's disease, which appear as enhancing nodules within the low-density mesenteric fat.
- Abscesses appear as low-density rim-enhancing fluid collections, in association with bowel wall and pericolic fat deposition, and are seen in Crohn's disease. Foci of low-density gas may be seen within the collections.
- Collections may fistulate into adjacent structures in Crohn's disease, resulting in enterovesical, enterocutaneous, perianal and rectovaginal fistulae. Fistulae are best

demonstrated in the presence of oral or rectal contrast; contrast-filled linear tracts may be seen extending to, or within, adjacent structures. Gas locules may be seen within these structures, confirming fistulation to a gas-containing viscus.

- Perforation is represented by a large collection of gas air in a non-dependent positions, i.e. the anterior part of the abdomen. Small locules of gas lying adjacent to inflamed bowel loops suggest the site of perforation. This is best appreciated on lung windows (Fig. 35.2).

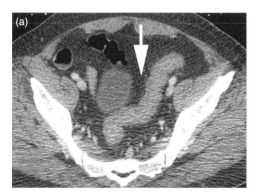

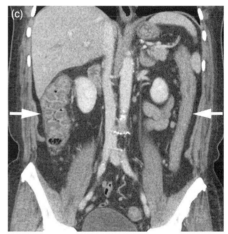

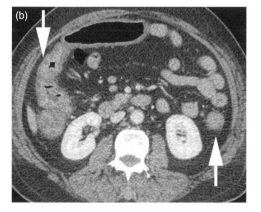

Fig. 35.1. (a), (b) Axial and (c) coronal images demonstrating diffuse pan-colonic wall thickening (arrows) consistent with ulcerative colitis.

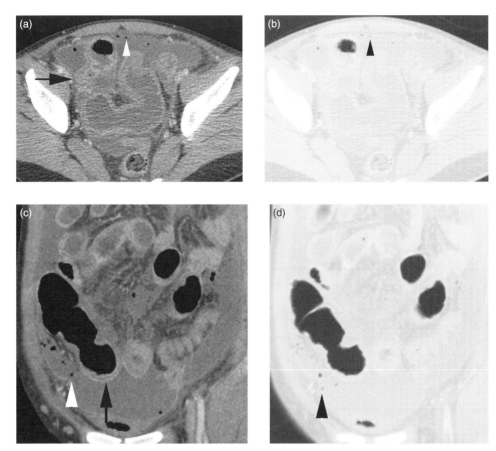

Fig. 35.2. Axial images on (a) soft tissue and (b) lung windows showing grossly inflamed distal small bowel and caecum in Crohn's colitis (black arrow). There is an adjacent fluid collection containing gas locules (arrowhead), suggestive of perforation. Coronal (c) soft tissue and (d) lung window images demonstrating the above findings.

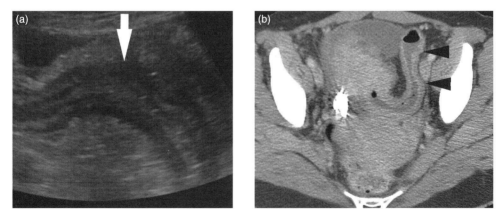

Fig. 35.3. (a) Longitudinal ultrasound image demonstrating diffuse wall thickening of the distal small bowel in the left iliac fossa (arrow). (b) Axial CT image in the same patient confirms the ultrasound finding of diffusely thickened distal small bowel (arrowhead), appearances are in keeping with Crohn's disease.

Ischaemic colitis

- Describes a group of clinical entities resulting from insufficient blood supply to segments of the entire colon, resulting in ischaemia.
- The resulting ischaemic necrosis ranges from mucosal involvement to mural/transmural involvement.
- Most commonly affects the left side of the colon, especially at the splenic flexure, where there is an arterial watershed between the superior and inferior mesenteric arterial territories. The rectum is usually spared.
- Results from diminished bowel perfusion secondary to low cardiac output, or occlusion of the bowel blood supply secondary to atheroma, thrombosis or embolism.
- Vasculitis, hypercoagulable states, bowel obstruction, trauma and pressor drugs, such as digitalis, have been linked.

Clinical features

- Presents with acute lower abdominal pain and tenderness, frequently located to the left side, and usually out of proportion to the clinical signs. There may be rectal bleeding or diarrhoea.
- In severe cases, bowel necrosis may result in perforation, and patients present with shock and peritonism.
- In mild cases, symptoms may resolve over several days with subsequent ischaemic stricture formation.

Radiological features

CT

- CT angiography allows the assessment of splanchnic vessels, namely the coeliac axis, superior and inferior mesenteric arteries. Low-density filling defects within an enhancing artery confirms the presence of thrombus. Reduced or non-enhancement suggests thrombosis or atherosclerotic narrowing.
- This should be followed by a portal venous phase study to assess bowel-wall enhancement and venous thrombosis.

Features

- The affected colon demonstrates symmetrical circumferential thickening with enlarged folds (Fig. 35.4). The bowel wall may demonstrate either low attenuation due to oedema, or high attenuation due to mural haemorrhage.
- Wall enhancement may be poor, with a sharp cut-off between normal and abnormal colon at the boundary of vascular territories.
- Mural gas, appearing as intramural locules of low attenuation, may be seen in severe disease, consistent with necrosis. In advanced disease, portal gas – appearing as branching low attenuation, usually in the left lobe of the liver – is a poor prognostic factor.

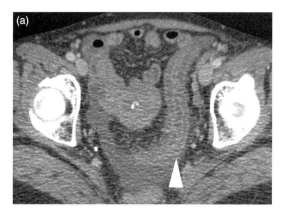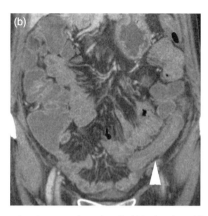

Fig. 35.4. (a) Axial and (b) coronal images showing diffusely thickened oedematous bowel wall within the sigmoid colon, with hyper-enhancement of the mucosa (arrowhead). The appearances are in keeping with ischaemic colitis. There is also a small amount of free fluid within the pelvis.

Pseudomembranous colitis

- This refers to the formation of a membranous exudate within the colon, identified with endoscopy; observed in approximately 50% of patients with this condition.

- *Clostridium difficile* is the primary causative pathogen, producing a toxin that results in an inflammatory reaction of the bowel wall.

- Affects 1 in 200 patients admitted to hospital: 25% will experience at least one recurrence.

- Predisposing factors include antibiotic exposure (including those used in its treatment), >65 years of age, chronic illness, altered gut motility, proton-pump inhibitors, chemotherapy agents, HIV infection and impaired immunity.

- Complications include toxic megacolon and perforation.

Clinical features

- Watery diarrhoea – up to 20 times per day, cramping abdominal pain, nausea, malaise and anorexia are common presentations.

- Fever and leucocytosis in acute infection.

- In severe cases, dehydration, hypotension, electrolyte disturbance and renal failure.

- Signs of peritonism may be present following perforation.

- Diagnosed by visualization of the pseudomembranes and stool assay for the toxin.

Radiological features

CT

Features

- Pathology primarily affects the mucosa and submucosa.
- Marked eccentric or circumferential wall thickening (Fig. 35.5), usually greater than in other forms of colitis, with the exception of Crohn's disease.
- Low density in the bowel wall suggests bowel-wall oedema.
- Significant enhancement due to bowel-wall hyperaemia.
- The *accordion sign* – trapping of oral contrast in between thickened haustral folds – is suggestive of severe pseudomembranous colitis.
- Ascites has been reported in up to 35% of patients, and can help differentiate between Crohn's disease and pseudomembranous colitis.

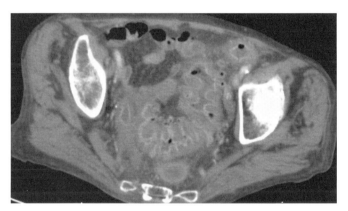

Fig. 35.5. Axial image showing marked circumferential sigmord colonic wall thickening with mucosial enhancement in keeping with pseudomembranous colitis.

Chapter

36

Diverticulitis

Characteristics

- Diverticul*osis*: focal herniation of the mucosa and submucosa through the muscular layer of the colon, at the natural openings for nutrient arteries.
- Diverticul*itis*: infection and inflammation of pre-existing diverticulosis caused by obstruction of the diverticula with faeces or undigested food material.
- The sigmoid colon has the highest intraluminal pressure and is therefore the commonest site of disease, although diverticulosis can occur anywhere along the length of the colon.
- Complications include perforation, with focal abscess formation, diverticular strictures – which can cause bowel obstruction – and colovesical and colovaginal fistula formation.

Clinical features

- Typically left iliac fossa pain, which may be associated with nausea, vomiting and bloating. Symptoms, however, will depend on the location of the diverticula.
- There may be raised inflammatory markers and pyrexia.
- In chronic diverticular disease, patients can present with a change in bowel habit, with alternating diarrhoea and constipation, large-bowel obstruction and blood/mucus per rectum.

Radiological features

CT

- Diverticula are seen as small outpouchings, containing gas or faeces, originating from the colonic wall.

Features
Acute diverticulitis

- Bowel-wall thickening, with inflammatory stranding in the adjacent fat.
- Hyperaemic bowel-wall enhancement.
- The presence of diverticula within the affected colonic segment confirms the diagnosis.

Complications

- A focal enhancing collection containing gas, adjacent to the affected segment, suggests a localized perforation (Fig. 36.1).

- Fistula formation to the bladder (colovesical) or vagina (colovaginal) may be inferred by the presence of air in these viscera. Rectal contrast may be useful in delineating the fistulous tract.

- Diverticular stricture formation, from chronic diverticular disease, may present with large-bowel obstruction.

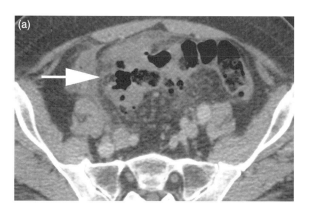

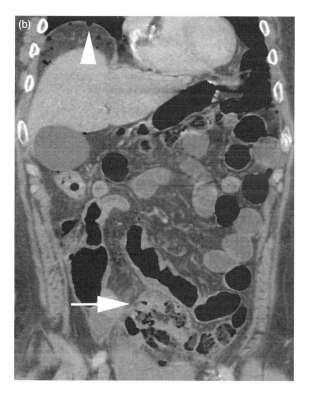

Fig. 36.1. (a) Axial and (b) coronal images showing bowel wall thickened within the sigmoid colon, with associated diverticular disease (arrow) and adjacent fatty inflammatory stranding. The appearance is in keeping with diverticulitis. Note also the free intra-abdominal gas locules secondary to perforation (arrowhead).

Chapter 37

Perforation

Characteristics

- Perforation of an air-containing hollow viscus allows free gas and/or fluid to enter the peritoneal cavity.
- Conditions most commonly complicated by perforation include duodenal ulcers, sigmoid diverticular disease, acute appendicitis and toxic megacolon.
- Small-bowel perforation is seen with trauma, foreign body ingestion, and with infiltrative disorders such as lymphoma.
- Pneumoperitoneum is common following laparoscopic/open surgery (up to 4 weeks post open surgery) or iatrogenic procedures such as drain insertions.

Clinical features

- Pain may initially be localized gradually becoming generalized secondary to peritonitis.
- Location of the pain may suggest the viscus involved. Upper abdominal pain suggests stomach or duodenum, whereas lower abdominal pain suggests colonic/pelvic pathology.
- On examination, tenderness and guarding may follow a similar pattern.
- Bowel sounds are reduced or absent with generalized peritonitis secondary to ileus.
- Be aware of the elderly patient who may present with vague symptoms and signs.

Radiological features

Plain radiographs

Erect chest x-ray (CXR)

- Sensitive method of demonstrating free sub-diaphragmatic air. Volumes as small as 1–2 ml of free air may be detected.
- Beware the supine patient elevated just prior to obtaining the erect film, as a short time interval is necessary for any gas to rise to a non-dependent position.

Right lateral decubitus abdominal x-ray (AXR)

- Useful if an erect CXR film cannot be obtained, or if the CXR findings are suspicious for a pneumoperitoneum.
- Gas (lucency) will outline the lateral edge of the liver.

AXR

- *Rigler's sign*: clearly delineated bowel wall due to the presence of gas on both sides of the bowel wall.
- Look for outlining of other intra-abdominal structures not usually well seen. These include the falciform ligament and the liver, diaphragmatic muscle slips, and lateral and medial umbilical ligaments.
- Diverticula, hernias, sub-diaphragmatic abscesses and chest pathology can all be mistaken for free air.
- *Chilaiditi syndrome*: colonic gas interposed between liver and diaphragm.

CT

Features

- The use of 'lung windows' increases the sensitivity for detecting free air, and is particularly invaluable in subtle cases.
- Look for free gas around the liver and upper abdomen (non-dependent).
- Look for locules of free gas adjacent to a suspected viscus (e.g. duodenum or sigmoid colon) (Fig. 36.1).
- Locules of free gas may be seen within free fluid, or contained fluid in the case of a sealed perforation.
- If gas is seen in the retroperitoneum, perforation of the 2nd to 4th parts of the duodenum (Fig. 37.1), ascending and descending colon, and rectum (Fig. 37.2) should be considered.

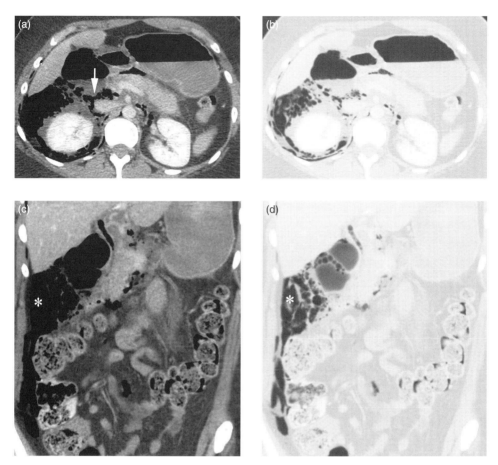

Fig. 37.1. Axial images on (a) soft tissue and (b) lung windows showing gas locules adjacent to the second part of the duodenum (arrow). Coronal images on (c) soft tissue and (d) lung windows demonstrating large-volume retroperitoneal gas (asterix). The study was performed following endoscopic retrograde cholangiopancreatography (ERCP). The appearances are in keeping with iatrogenic duodenal perforation.

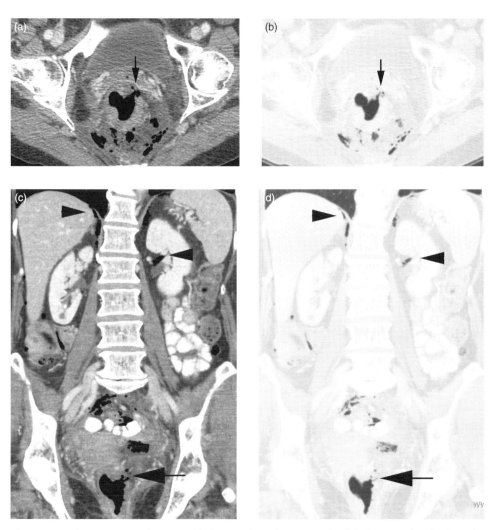

Fig. 37.2. Axial images on (a) soft tissue and (b) lung windows showing rectal wall thickening and gas locules in the mesorectal fat (black arrow). Coronal images on (c) soft tissue and (d) lung windows showing intraperitoneal and retroperitoneal gas locules (black arrowheads). The study was performed following transanal endoscopic microsurgery (TEMS). The appearances are in keeping with iatrogenic rectal perforation.

Chapter 38

Renal tract calculi

Characteristics

- There is a male preponderance; the M:F ratio is 3:1.
- Three common sites of renal tract obstruction: the pelvi-ureteric junction (PUJ), the pelvic brim and the vesico-ureteric junction (VUJ).
- Causes of renal tract calculi include chronically raised levels of calcium excretion, abnormalities in oxalate, cystine, urate and xanthine metabolism, urological sepsis, urinary stagnation and chronic dehydration.
- The four main types of renal calculi are calcium (75%), struvite (15%), uric acid (6%) and cystine (2%).
- Antiretroviral medications, such as protease inhibitors, classically cause renal tract calculi that are not visible on a CT scan.
- Renal calculi predispose to infection. If left untreated, obstruction – in association with infection – can cause pyonephrosis, perinephric abscess formation and urosepsis.

Clinical features

- Severe colicky abdominal pain classically radiating from loin to groin in a 'restless' patient. The pain is often described as 'worse than labour', and can be associated with nausea and vomiting.
- Haematuria is usually present but may only be identifiable on a urine dipstick.

Radiological features

- 90% of renal tract calculi may be radio-opaque on plain radiography.

Ultrasound

- Point-of-care ultrasound is increasingly being used, and is an extremely useful diagnostic aid in the emergency setting.
- Depending on local protocol, it can be used as a discharge tool in pain-controlled young patients with no signs of obstruction. A comparison of ureteric jets in the bladder is aided by colour or power Doppler to confirm dynamic ureteric function (Fig. 38.1).
- In the elderly population it can be used to exclude an abdominal aortic aneurysm.

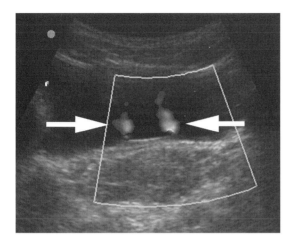

Fig. 38.1. Duplex ultrasound image demonstrating presence of bilateral ureteric jets (arrows).

CT

- Low-dose CT scan performed without contrast.
- Patients should have a full bladder and scanned in a prone position. This allow VUJ stones to be distinguished from dependent bladder calculi.

Features

- Follow the ureters from renal pelvis to bladder on each side. Renal tract calcification is easily identifiable as high-density foci. Knowledge of the ureteric course will help distinguish renal calculi from calcification within adjacent structures, e.g. arterial, venous (phlebolith), nodal and prostatic.
- Ureteric wall thickening may be seen surrounding a high-density ureteric calculus, known as the *tissue rim sign*.
- Secondary signs of urinary obstruction/inflammation include the following.
  - An enlarged kidney with slightly decreased attenuation, due to oedema. A >5 HU density difference compared with the opposite non-obstructed kidney is thought to be significant.
  - Perinephric and periureteric fat stranding, secondary to oedema.
  - A mildly dilated pelvicalyceal system is suggestive of acute obstruction (comparison with the opposite non-obstructed kidney is often useful) (Fig. 38.2).
  - Severe pelvicalyceal dilatation is more in keeping with a chronically dilated system.
  - Forniceal rupture, secondary to urinary obstruction, may cause focal perinephric collections.
  - Gas seen within the collecting system is highly suggestive of a pyonephrosis. This is a urological emergency which requires urgent nephrostomy drainage.

- Common pitfalls
  - An extrarenal pelvis and parapelvic cysts may be misinterpreted as hydronephrosis.
  - Atherosclerotic calcification may be misinterpreted as ureteric calculi.
  - Phleboliths are well-defined round areas of calcification found within the pelvic veins, which can be mistaken for renal tract calculi. They characteristically have a central lucency, and may demonstrate a *tail sign*, which is a tail of non-calcified vein extending from the phlebolith.

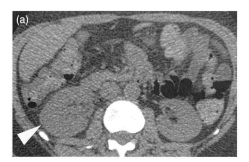

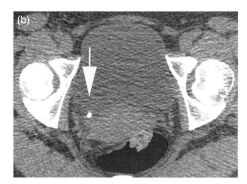

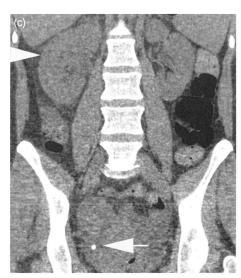

Fig. 38.2. (a), (b) Axial and (c) coronal images showing swollen right kidney and hydronephrosis (arrowhead) secondary to right VUJ calculi (arrow).

Chapter

39

Intussusception

Characteristics

- Invagination or prolapse of a segment of intestinal tract (= *intussusceptum*) into the lumen of the adjacent distal intestine (= *intussuscipiens*).
- 90% are ileocolic and ileo-ileocolic.

Adult intussusception

- The majority arise from a pathological lead point.
- Causes include lipomas, carcinomas, metastases and lymphoma.

Paediatric intussusception

- 90% of all paediatric intussusceptions have no pathological lead point and are thought to be associated with lymphoid hyperplasia in Peyer's patches of the ileum.
- 10% have a lead point, which include a Meckel's diverticulum, polyps or other tumours, and duplication cysts.
- Intussusception usually occurs within the first 2 years, and rarely in neonates.

Clinical features

- The patient presents with severe colicky pain and vomiting. Initial stools passed at the start of symptoms are unremarkable; blood and mucus ('redcurrant jelly') stools are passed after 24 hours.
- On examination, there may be a palpable sausage-shaped mass, most often in the upper abdomen.

Radiological features

Ultrasound

- The modality of choice in paediatric patients.

Features

- A mass is usually demonstrated in the right upper quadrant, adjacent to the gallbladder, in ileocolic intussusceptions, which are the most common type in paediatric patients. A full abdominal scan should be performed, as an intussusception can occur anywhere.

- Transverse section through the 'mass' reveals concentric alternating hyperechoic and hypoechoic rings, representing compressed mucosal and serosal surfaces and oedematous bowel wall, respectively (*target/doughnut sign*) (Figs. 39.1 and 39.2a).

- A longitudinal section through the mass demonstrates a hypoechoic mass with an appearance very similar to a kidney (*pseudo-kidney sign*) (Fig. 39.2b). It is essential that the right kidney is seen separately from this to prevent a false positive result.

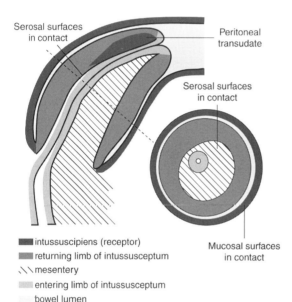

Serosal surfaces in contact

Peritoneal transudate

Serosal surfaces in contact

Mucosal surfaces in contact

▆▆ intussuscipiens (receptor)
▆▆ returning limb of intussusceptum
╲╲ mesentery
░░ entering limb of intussusceptum
bowel lumen

Fig. 39.1. Line drawing demonstrating the relationship of the intussusceptum and intussuscipiens.

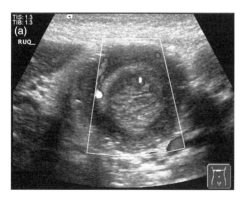
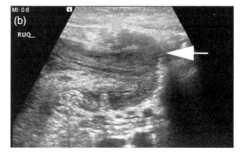

Fig. 39.2. (a) Transverse ultrasound image of an intussusception, demonstrating alternating hyperechoic and hypoechoic rings, consistent with the *doughnut sign*.
(b) Longitudinal ultrasound image demonstrating *pseudo-kidney* appearance of the intussusception (arrow).

- Occasionally, a lymph node or tumour mass may be seen within the intussusceptum, the lead point for the intussusception.
- Increased flow is demonstrated on colour Doppler due to blood vessels within the mesentery, which have been dragged in between the entering and exiting layers of the intussusception (Fig. 39.2a). An absence of blood flow is suggestive of bowel ischaemia/necrosis.
- Free fluid may be present but is non-specific.

CT

Features

- The intussuscipiens is markedly dilated and contains an eccentric soft-tissue intussusceptum.
- The intussusceptum brings the mesentery and associated blood vessels with it into the

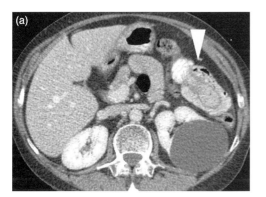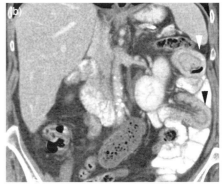

Fig. 39.3. (a) Axial and (b) coronal images demonstrating the intussuscipiens and intussusceptum, with its associated low-attenuation mesentery and in-drawn vessels (arrowheads).

intussuscipiens. This is demonstrated by low-density fat tissue and in-drawing of linear enhancing vessels (Fig. 39.3). A lead point may be demonstrated at the apex of the intussusceptum.

Radiological management

Paediatric intussusception only

- An intussusception can be reduced radiologically under fluoroscopic guidance with barium, water-soluble contrast or air, in a fluid-resuscitated patient. This should be performed by a paediatric radiologist, with paediatric surgical support.
- Contraindications to fluoroscopic intervention include pneumoperitoneum and peritonitis.

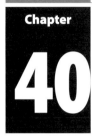

Chapter

40

Pancreatitis

Characteristics

- Acute inflammation damages the acinar tissue and small ducts of the pancreas, allowing pancreatic secretions to escape easily due to the absence of a pancreatic capsule.
- Pancreatic enzymes are rapidly distributed to different anatomical compartments by digesting through fascial layers.
- 80% of cases occur secondary to cholelithiasis or alcohol excess.
- 10% of cases are idiopathic.
- Chronic pancreatitis, for which alcohol excess is responsible in 70% of cases, causes progressive damage to the pancreatic tissue, with irreversible fibrosis.

Clinical features

- Patients classically present with epigastric pain, which radiates to the back, associated with nausea and vomiting.
- In acute severe pancreatitis, there may be profound systemic upset including shock, adult respiratory distress syndrome (ARDS), multi-organ failure, flank ecchymosis (*Grey–Turner sign*) and periumbilical ecchymosis (*Cullen sign*).

Radiological features

Ultrasound

Features
- Enlarged hypoechoic gland, caused by diffuse oedema.
- The pancreatic duct may be dilated.
- Complications of acute pancreatitis may be evident (see below).

CT

- Triple-phase scan performed, comprising unenhanced scan, to show evidence of pancreatic calcification, supplemented by arterial and portal venous phase scans.

- Acute pancreatitis is a clinical diagnosis. CT is performed to assess for the presence and severity of complications.

Features
Acute pancreatitis

- Enlarged pancreas of reduced attenuation, with an indistinct contour due to oedema (Fig. 40.1).
- Inflammatory stranding in the adjacent peripancreatic fat.
- Thickening of the lateral conal fascia and Gerota's fascia.

Chronic pancreatitis

- Coarse or spiculated pancreatic calcification.
- Dilated pancreatic duct (>5 mm in the head of the pancreas, >2mm in the body).

Complications

Fluid collection: Low-attenuation, homogeneous, non-encapsulated fluid within the pancreatic bed and retroperitonuem, outlining fascial planes.

Pancreatic necrosis: Areas of non-enhancing parenchyma due to pancreatic necrosis (Fig. 40.2).

Haemorrhage: Autodigestion of blood vessels by pancreatic enzymes may result in high-density (>50 HU) haemorrhage into the peritoneal cavity or retroperitoneum.

Pseudocysts: Well-defined oval fluid collection surrounded by a fibrous capsule; develops 6 weeks following acute pancreatitis.

Pseudoaneurysms: Saccular outpouching of an eroded artery, most commonly involves the splenic artery. The fragility of the pseudoaneurysm wall increases risk of rupture and life-threatening haemorrhage.

Venous thrombosis: The inflammatory process results in increased risk of thrombosis in adjacent veins, including the splenic and renal veins. Thrombus is seen as low-attenuation filling defects within the lumen of the vein, on portal venous phase imaging.

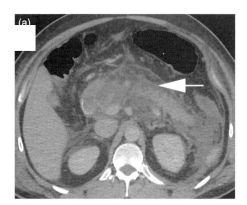 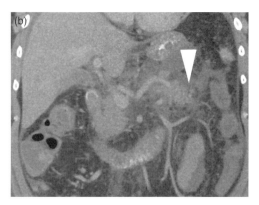

Fig. 40.1. (a) Axial and (b) coronal images demonstrating pancreatic oedema, with stranding in the adjacent mesenteric fat, consistent with acute pancreatitis (arrow and arrowhead).

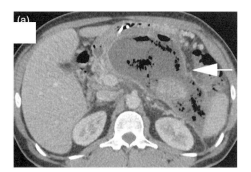 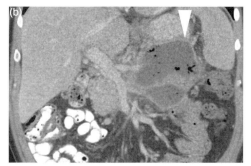

Fig. 40.2. (a) Axial and (b) coronal images demonstrating advanced pancreatitis, complicated by necrosis. A large enhancing collection, containing fluid and gas locules, has replaced the pancreatic parenchyma (arrow and arrowhead).

Chapter

41

Testicular torsion

Characteristics

- Torsion or twisting of the spermatic cord causes strangulation of the gonadal blood supply resulting in testicular ischaemia and necrosis.
- Torsion is a urological emergency that requires urgent surgical treatment.
- There are two common types of torsion.

  Extravaginal torsion

  o Occurs in the neonatal period before the testes have descended fully into the scrotum.

  o Develops prenatally in the spermatic cord proximal to the tunica vaginalis attachment.

  o 70% occur prenatally, 30% occur postnatally.

  Intravaginal torsion

  o Occurs in older children due to a congenital anomaly known as the 'bell clapper deformity'.

  o This anomaly results in an abnormally high attachment of the tunica vaginalis to the testicle.

  o The long axis of the testicle is then orientated transversely, allowing the testicle to rotate spontaneously on the spermatic cord.

  o The bell clapper deformity is found in 12% of males; in 40% of these individuals the anomaly will be bilateral.

Clinical features

- Patients present with sudden onset of severe unilateral testicular pain and scrotal swelling. Often associated with nausea and vomiting.
- A previous history of similar testicular pain, which resolves without treatment, is suggestive of intermittent torsion with spontaneous resolution.

Radiological features

Ultrasound

- Testicular torsion is a clinical diagnosis and should be referred to urology for appropriate surgical management without delay.
- In equivocal cases, ultrasound may help to exclude other possible diagnoses.
- Both testes should be imaged and compared.

Features

Normal testes
- Similar sized testicles.
- Homogeneous, symmetrical echotexture.
- Colour Doppler flow in the testes and epididymides should be equal.

Testicular torsion
- Testicular enlargement.
- Uniformly hypoechoic echotexture (early) (Fig. 41.1).
- Heterogeneous echotexture indicating areas of necrosis (late).
- Colour Doppler flow may be absent (late) or normal/increased due to spontaneous resolution (Fig. 41.2).

Epididymo-orchitis
- Testicular and epididymal enlargement.
- Heterogeneous echotexture.
- Colour Doppler flow in the testis and epididymis are increased.

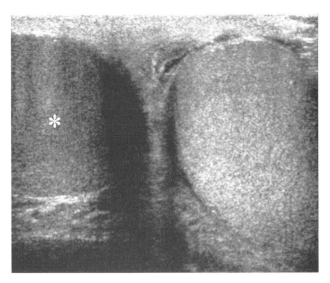

Fig. 41.1. Transverse ultrasound image demonstrating reduced echogenicity of the right testis (asterix) compared with the contralateral side.

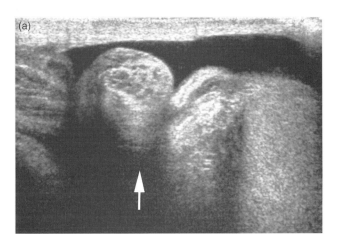

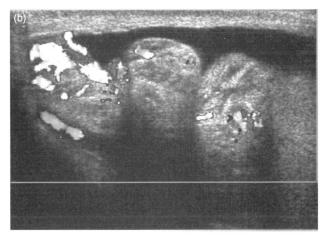

Fig. 41.2. Longitudinal images demonstrating (a) twisting of the spermatic cord in keeping with testicular torsion (arrow); (b) increased vascularity, which may be seen with torsion. A small hydrocele is also present surrounding the right testis.

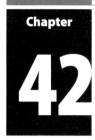

Chapter

Ectopic pregnancy

Characteristics

- Derived from the Greek word *ektopos*, meaning 'out of place'.

- Describes the implantation of a fertilized egg in a location other than the endometrial lining of the uterus. 95% occur in the ampullary or isthmic portion of the fallopian tubes.

- Occurs in 2% of pregnancies and accounts for 9% of all pregnancy-related deaths, second only to venous thromboembolism.

- Many factors increase the risk of ectopic pregnancy, by affecting the migration of the embryo to the endometrial cavity.

- Risk factors include pelvic inflammatory disease, most commonly caused by *Chlamydia trachomatis*, previous history of ectopic pregnancy, prior tubal surgery, fertility drugs/ assisted reproductive technology, intra-uterine contraceptive devices, age >35 years and smoking.

- Usually presents by 7th week of pregnancy.

- High index of suspicion is required as symptoms are similar to other common conditions: appendicitis, salpingitis, ruptured corpus luteum cyst, spontaneous abortion, ovarian torsion and urinary tract disease. Missed or delayed diagnosis can be devastating, with massive haemorrhage and possibly death.

Clinical features

- Classical triad of lower abdominal pain, amenorrhoea, and vaginal bleeding is seen in 50% of patients.

- Patients may present with symptoms of early pregnancy: nausea, breast fullness, fatigue, low abdominal pain, heavy cramping, shoulder pain and recent dyspareunia.

- Findings of haemorrhagic shock, including hypotension and tachycardia, may be absent due to the physiological changes of pregnancy.

- Other findings to support an ectopic pregnancy include adnexal tenderness/mass and peritonism following rupture.

Radiological features

Ultrasound

- The imaging modality of choice, which can either be performed transabdominally or transvaginally. The latter is more sensitive, whereas the former is less invasive.

Features

- An extra-uterine sac containing a fetal pole or yolk sac, with or without cardiac motion, is observed in <20% of cases and confirms an ectopic pregnancy (Fig. 42.1).

- A thick-walled cystic structure or a complex adnexal mass, independent of the ovary and uterus, is also suggestive of ectopic pregnancy.

- Identification of a viable intra-uterine gestation sac virtually rules out an ectopic pregnancy, except in the rare circumstance of a heterotopic pregnancy (incidence of 1 in 7,000 pregnancies) (Fig. 42.2).

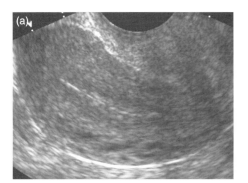
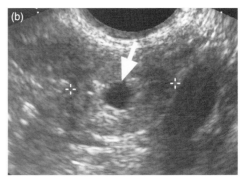

Fig. 42.1. Longitudinal images demonstrating (a) a normal uterus with no intra-uterine pregnancy identified, (b) an exta-uterine gestation sac within the right adnexa (arrow).

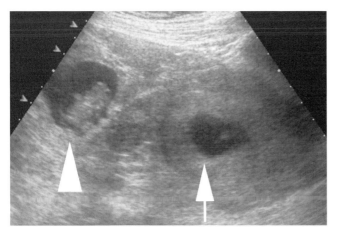

Fig. 42.2. Heterotopic pregnancy: transverse image showing a normal intra-uterine gestational sac (arrow). There is an additional extra-uterine gestational sac containing a viable foetus (arrowhead).

- Other supportive findings include absence of an intra-uterine pregnancy at 6 weeks gestation, pelvic free fluid or hyperechoic clot within the uterus, hydro- or haematosalpinx or a thickened endometrium. A pseudogestational sac may be seen, consisting of endometrial thickening with an anechoic centre composed of haemorrhage. This is classically 'teardrop' in shape and should not be confused with an intra-uterine pregnancy (Fig. 42.3).

- In cases of rupture, extensive anechoic intra-abdominal and pelvic haemorrhage may be seen. This can also be seen on CT (Fig. 42.4), although this is not routinely performed due to the potential risks of ionizing radiation.

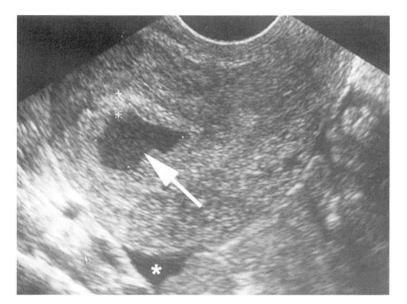

Fig. 42.3. Transvaginal image showing a teardrop-shaped pseudogestational sac. Free fluid is seen within the pouch of Douglas (asterix).

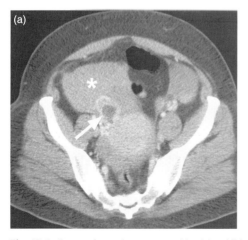
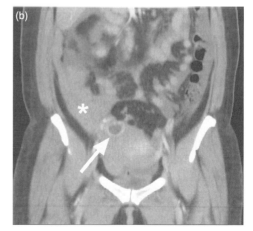

Fig. 42.4. Ruptured ectopic pregnancy: (a) axial and (b) coronal images demonstrating an extra-uterine gestational sac (arrow) with extensive haemoperitonium (asterix).

Chapter

43

Ovarian cyst/torsion

Characteristics

Ovarian cyst

- Defined as a fluid-filled sac within the ovary.
- Commonest in women of childbearing age, but can affect women of all ages.
- Diagnosis has become more frequent with the wider application of ultrasound.
- The majority of cysts are considered functional and remain asymptomatic.
- Symptoms described include lower abdominal pain, bloating, irregular menstrual cycle and dyspareunia.
- Complications are uncommon and include rupture, torsion and haemorrhage into a cyst.

Ovarian torsion

- Torsion of the ovary is the fifth most common gynaecological emergency, accounting for 3% of all gynaecological emergencies.
- Risk factors include enlarged ovaries >6 cm, elongated ovarian ligaments, and strenuous exercise.
- Caused by twisting of the vascular pedicle with associated venous or arterial occlusion and subsequent infarction.
- Patients typically present with abdominal pain, nausea and vomiting. Fever is classically associated with tissue necrosis.
- Long-term complications such as infertility and premature menopause have been reported.
- Early diagnosis facilitates laparoscopic intervention without the complications of traditional open surgery.

Radiological features

Ultrasound

- Transabdominal scanning with a full bladder is generally well tolerated. Transvaginal scanning, while representing the 'gold standard', is less patient-friendly and requires appropriate training and an endocavity probe.

Features

- A thin-walled anechoic structure in the adnexa >2.5 cm is consistent with an ovarian cyst (Fig. 43.1a). Internal echogenicity demonstrating movement suggests haemorrhage (Fig. 43.1b). Most cysts <5 cm are asymptomatic and should not be assumed to be the cause of the patient's presentation.

- A cyst with septations, solid components and increased vascularity on Doppler scanning is suspicious of malignancy (Fig. 43.1c).

- Free fluid seen within the abdomen is suggestive of cyst rupture. In the absence of a visible cyst, a review of previous ultrasound studies may be useful.

- Torsion is characterized by an oedematous ovary, typically enlarged, with reduced or absent Doppler signal on Duplex.

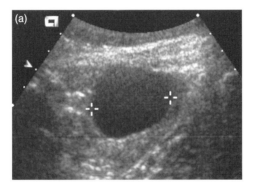

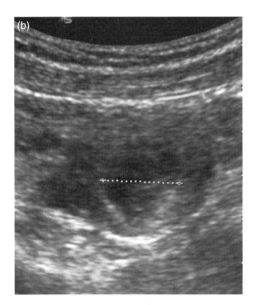
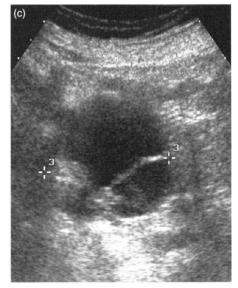

Fig. 43.1. Ultrasound images of the ovary, demonstrating (a) an anechoic simple cyst, (b) a hypoechoic cyst with internal echoes, consistent with a haemorrhagic cyst, and (c) a complex cyst containing both fluid and solid components suspicious for malignancy.

Irritable hip/transient synovitis

Characteristics

- Defined as transient inflammation of the synovium of the hip.
- The most common cause of non-traumatic hip pain.
- Affects children aged 4–10 years, with twice as many boys than girls affected.
- Vital to exclude septic arthritis, which can lead to significant joint destruction. Particularly important in patients with haemophilia or immunocompromised patients, such as those with HIV, sickle cell anaemia or secondary to chemotherapy treatment.
- 1.5% of patients develop *Legg–Calvé–Perthes* disease, resulting in avascular necrosis of the femoral head; thought to be related to increased intra-articular pressure, although this association remains controversial.
- Recent history of upper respiratory tract infection may be identified in approximately half the patients.

Clinical features

- Unilateral hip or groin pain is the most common complaint.
- Crying and an antalgic limp may be the only observation in very young children.
- Pseudo-paralysis may be seen on examination. This is when the child orientates the joint in flexion, abduction and external rotation in order to minimize pain, and resists passive movement.
- Swelling and oedema are difficult to detect, as the hip joint is too deep to palpate. Pain may be elicited on passive movement.
- Onset may be sudden or gradual, with spontaneous recovery after several days.

Radiological features

Ultrasound

- The imaging of choice, with >95% sensitivity. Effusions are rarely detectable on plain radiographs.
- A high-frequency linear probe should be used.

Features

- If a joint effusion is present, an anechoic collection is seen superficial to the echogenic cortex of the femur (Fig. 44.1).

- It is common to mistake synovial thickening for collections. This is best differentiated with the use of colour Doppler, where increased colour flow is seen in synovial thickening, compared with the absence of flow within fluid collections. Fluid collections may also be compressible, helping to differentiate from synovial thickening.

- Asymmetry of fluid depth between the two hip joints of >3 mm confirms the presence of a pathological joint effusion.

- Ultrasound cannot differentiate between a simple effusion, pus and haemorrhage.

- Aspiration under ultrasound guidance should be performed if there are signs suggestive of septic arthritis. This should be performed in close liaison with paediatricians.

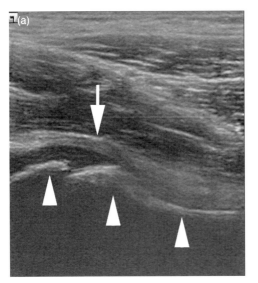 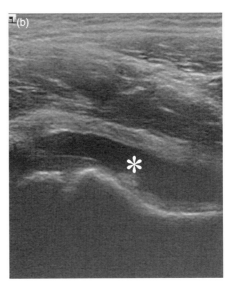

Fig. 44.1. a) Longitudinal image of the normal right hip joint with joint capsule (arrow) closely related to the echogenic femoral cortex (arrowheads). b) Longitudinal image of left hip containing joint effussion (asterix) with bulging of the joint capsule.

Chapter

45

Knee soft-tissue injury

Characteristics

- A common injury usually following a discrete episode of trauma (twisting injury, side-stepping, sports tackle injury, high-energy road traffic collision).
- The mechanism of injury can help to localize and predict the injury pattern, e.g. a rapid deceleration injury or posterior force on the proximal tibia is associated with a posterior cruciate ligament (PCL) injury.
- May lead to significant knee instability; therefore it is important to recognize the injury early and treat appropriately.
- If left untreated, can lead to secondary osteoarthritis and immobility.

Clinical features

- Pain exacerbated by movement, swelling of the knee and an inability to bear weight.
- Patients may report a 'snap' or 'pop' at the time of injury.
- A history of locking, or the knee 'giving way', is significant.
- The following examination tests can help in the assessment for particular injuries.
    - *Lachman test* – to assess anterior cruciate ligament (ACL) laxity.
    - *Straight-leg raise* – to assess quadriceps and patella tendon rupture.

Radiological features

MRI

- The 'gold standard' for assessing soft-tissue injuries, as it provides excellent soft-tissue contrast.
- High negative predictive value; thus a normal scan virtually excludes internal derangement.
- Identifies those patients requiring invasive arthroscopy.

Features

Anterior cruciate ligament (ACL) injury

- A mid-substance tear is the most common site of injury.

- Non-visualization, or discontinuity, of the fibres of the ACL (Fig. 45.1).

- Associated microtrabecular fractures (high signal on STIR/T2W images) within the lateral femoral condyle and posterolateral tibial plateau.

- Associated anterior tibial translation.

- Common associated injuries include:

  o Medial menicus tear

  o Medial collateral ligament tear

  o Segond fracture – avulsion fracture of the lateral tibial condyle.

Medial collateral ligament (MCL) injury

- The MCL is closely related to the medial joint capsule and medial meniscus.

- High signal within, and surrounding, the ligament indicates an injury.

- Can be associated with meniscocapsular separation, where high-signal fluid is seen between the medial meniscus and the capsule.

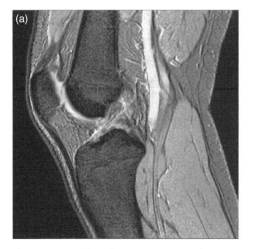
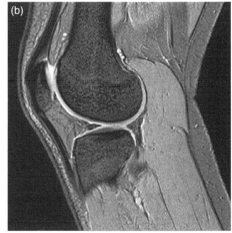

Fig. 45.1. Sagittal gradient T2W images: (a) demonstrating discontinuity and increased signal within the fibres of the ACL, consistent with a rupture; (b) demonstrating associated anterior tibial translation (a vertical line drawn from the posterior border of the femoral condyle should lie within 5 mm of the posterior cortex of the adjacent tibia).

Meniscal injury

- High signal within a meniscus, extending to an articular surface, indicates a tear; this may be horizontal or vertical (Fig. 45.2).
- In a 'bucket-handle' meniscal tear, the torn meniscus may be visible within the intercondylar notch, referred to as the *double PCL sign* (Fig. 45.3).

Extensor mechanism injury

- Altered signal and/or discontinuity within the quadriceps or patellar tendons (Fig. 45.4).

Posterior cruciate ligament injury

- Discontinuity in the fibres of the PCL.
- Associated posterior tibial translation.
- Not usually associated with knee instability.

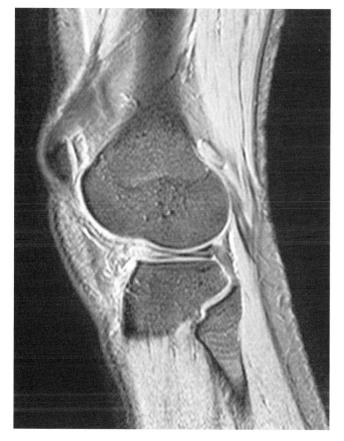

Fig. 45.2. Sagittal gradient T2 image demonstrating horizontal high signal within the meniscus extending to the superior articular surface, consistent with a horizontal cleavage tear. There is also high signal in the anterior portion of the meniscus.

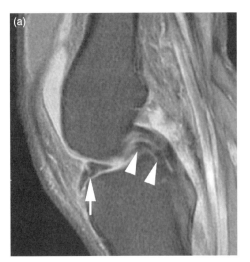

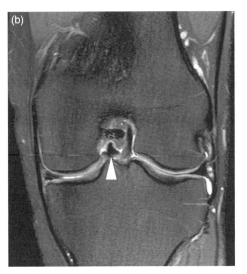

Fig. 45.3. (a) Sagittal gradient T2W image demonstrating the *double PCL sign* (arrowheads) consistent with a bucket-handle tear of the medial meniscus. Notes also the linear high signal within the medial meniscus anteriorly related to the tear (arrow). (b) Coronal gradient T2W image demonstrating low-signal fragment within the intercondylar notch from the flipped bucket-handle meniscal fragment (arrowhead).

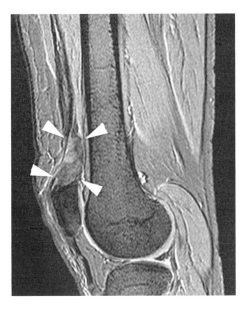

Fig. 45.4. Sagittal gradient T2W image demonstrating high signal within the quadriceps tendon consistent with rupture (arrowheads).

Chapter 46

Achilles tendon rupture

Characteristics

- The Achilles tendon is the largest and strongest tendon in the body.
- Formed from the tendinous portions of the gastrocnemius and soleus muscles, converging 15 cm proximal to its insertion at the posterior calcaneus.
- The *watershed zone*, approximately 2–6 cm proximal to the calcaneus, is the most common site of degeneration and rupture. This is thought to be due to the sparse blood supply in this region that occurs with progressive aging.
- Rupture occurs most commonly in men between 30 and 50 years old, and may be partial or complete.
- Risk factors include increase in physical activity, corticosteroid injection and previous rupture.
- The most common mechanism of injury follows sudden forced plantar flexion with contraction of the gastrocnemius-soleus. Patients classically report a sensation of being kicked in the back of the leg, followed by severe pain.
- There is a spectrum of other Achilles tendon injuries including: peritenonitis, tendinosis with peritenonitis, and tendinosis, representing progressive stages of injury.

Clinical features

- Related to the stage of injury:
  - Peritenonitis – localized burning pain tracking along the Achilles tendon following activity.
  - Tendinosis with peritenonitis – nodular thickening may be present. Activity-related pain, swelling and crepitation along the tendon sheath.
  - Tendinosis – final stage with focal and nodular thickening in the posterior aspect of the tendon. No pain is reported, due to the lack of inflammation.
- Rupture usually presents with a sudden snapping sensation in the back of the leg followed by severe pain. Patients usually remain mobile but are unable to run, climb stairs or stand on tiptoe, due to loss of plantar flexion.

- A palpable gap may be detected on examination along with other signs:
  - *Hyper-dorsiflexion sign* – The patient lies prone with the knee flexed. Excessive dorsiflexion of the affected side results, with passive flexion of the foot.
  - *Simmonds–Thompson test* – squeezing of the calf while the patient is lying prone with their feet hanging off the end of the bed. Lack of plantar flexion is a positive sign consistent with rupture.

Radiological features

Ultrasound

- The imaging of choice in the acute setting to evaluate a suspected rupture. Diagnosis of all three stages of Achilles tendon injuries can also be made on MRI.

Features

- Normal tendons have a thickness of <7 mm and uniform echogenicity (Fig. 46.1).
- Fusiform swelling with heterogeneous echotexture, and focal hypoechogenicity (mucoid degeneration) are consistent with tendinosis (Fig. 46.2).

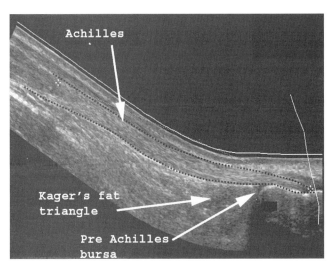

Fig. 46.1. Longitudinal ultrasound image demonstrating the appearance of a normal Achilles tendon.

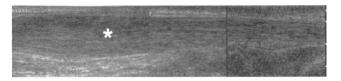

Fig. 46.2. Longitudinal ultrasound image showing fusiform swelling of the proximal Achilles tendon (asterix), in keeping with Achilles tendinopathy.

- Loss of tendinous continuity, denoted by an area of reduced echogenicity, suggests rupture. However, the tendon gap is often replaced with haematoma, which may appear echogenic (Fig. 46.3).

- Confirmation of rupture is best demonstrated on dynamic scanning of the tendon during passive movement. In complete rupture, the proximal portion of the ruptured tendon will not slide on passive plantar flexion.

- Partial rupture can also be diagnosed using this technique, as part of the tendon may still demonstrate sliding on dynamic assessment, despite the apparent loss of tendon continuity.

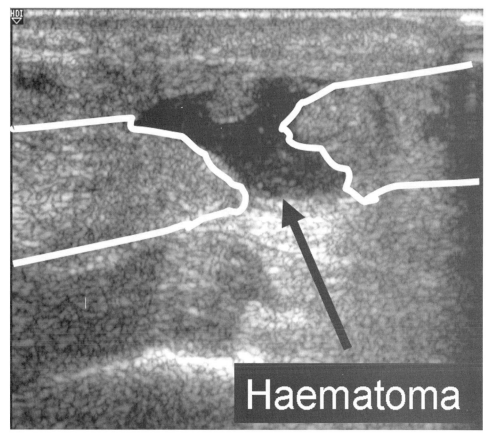

Fig. 46.3. Longitudinal ultrasound image demonstrating complete rupture of the Achilles tendon. There is a gap between the two ends of the ruptured tendon with reduced echogenicity consistent with haematoma.

Chapter

47

Discitis

Characteristics

- Inflammation of an intervertebral disc, usually associated with infection (pure discitis).
- More commonly, infection is present within the adjacent vertebral body (osteomyelitis) and then spreads into the disc rather than vice versa. However, in primary discitis, the adjacent vertebral end-plates are rapidly destroyed.
- The lumbar spine is most commonly affected, followed by the cervical and thoracic spines.
- The intervertebral disc obtains its nutrients from the vertebral end-plates, which are supplied by end-arteries. Septic emboli can travel to these end-arteries causing end-plate infarction. Localized infection then rapidly spreads through the vertebral body and enters the intervertebral disc.
- Haematogenous infection can spread to vertebral bodies from distant sites, including the pelvis (most commonly), chest and soft tissues. Osteomyelitis (vertebritis) (Fig. 2.8) can also occur secondary to spinal procedures (including spinal or epidural injections).
- The most common causative organism is *Staphylococcus aureus* (50–60%). Other causal organisms include Gram-negative organisms, particularly *E. coli*, *Proteus* and *Pseudomonas* (intravenous drug abuse).
- Direct spread of infection is often iatrogenic (discography, chemonucleolysis or discectomy).
- In immunocompromised patients, opportunistic pathogens must be suspected, including tuberculosis (TB).
- Pott's disease – vertebral body and disc involvement with TB (non-pyogenic):
  - Commonly involves the thoracic spine
  - Bone destruction is considerable
  - Multiple vertebrae affected, with relative sparing of the intervening discs
  - Spreads beneath the anterior longitudinal ligament causing anterior vertebral irregularity and Gibbus deformity
  - Large paraspinal abscesses are common.

Clinical features

- History of an antecedent invasive procedure (direct spread) or a recent systemic infection (secondary discitis/osteomyelitis).
- Insidious onset can delay diagnosis. Back pain, localized to a particular spinal segment, aggravated by movement and not relieved with analgesia.
- Spinal infection can track down muscle planes, causing muscle spasm, or can present as groin or buttock abscesses.
- Mild pyrexia or tachycardia with raised inflammatory markers. The relevant spinal segment is usually tender to palpation.
- Complications include epidural abscess and paravertebral soft-tissue masses.

Radiological features

CT

Features

- Disc space narrowing, hypodense intervertebral disc and destruction of the adjacent end-plates.
- Paravertebral soft-tissue mass with extension into the epidural space.
- Radiological guided biopsy is essential for accurate microbiological assessment.

MRI

- The imaging modality of choice, with 95% accuracy.

Features

- Decreased marrow signal in two contiguous vertebral end-plates and intervening disc, with blurring of the margins on T1W (due to oedema) (Fig. 47.1).
- Increased marrow signal in two contiguous vertebrae and intervening disc on T2W (due to oedema, infarction or abscess) (Fig. 47.1b).
- Paraspinal/epidural abscess: isointense on T1, hyperintense on T2, and STIR.
- Contrast enhancement in the end-plates, intervening disc and paraspinal/epidural abscess.

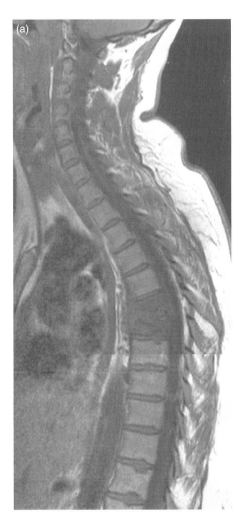
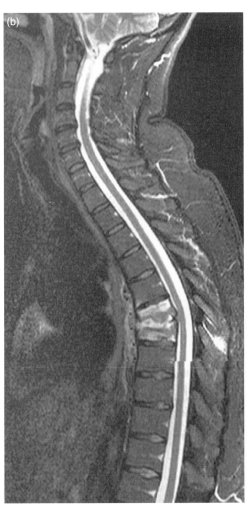

Fig. 47.1. Sagittal (a) T1W and (b) STIR MRI images of the cervicothoracic spine, demonstrating low T1 signal and corresponding high signal on STIR of the T6 and T7 vertebral bodies and intervening disc. There is also evidence of vertebral body collapse secondary to bony destruction. Appearances are in keeping with discitis, with destruction of the adjacent end-plates.

Chapter

48

Prolapsed intervertebral disc/Cauda equina syndrome

Characteristics

- An intervertebral disc consists of a central nucleus pulposus, bound by an annulus fibrosus. Herniation of the disc material (nucleus) through the posterior longitudinal ligament can cause irritation or compression of the nerve roots within or exiting the central canal, resulting in a radiculopathy or sciatica.

- A lifetime prevalence of back pain is between 50% and 80%; however, only 5% of males and 2.5% of females will experience a radiculopathy.

- Disc prolapses most commonly occur at L4/5 and L5/S1, with L5 radiculopathy being most commonly found in clinical practice.

- The cauda equina represents the nerve roots sited caudal to the level of the spinal cord termination (conus). Compression of these nerve roots leads to cauda equina syndrome, producing symptoms of unilateral or bilateral sciatica, saddle sensory anaesthesia, bladder and bowel dysfunction, in addition to lower back pain.

- Compression of the cauda equina can be secondary to trauma, disc prolapses, abscesses, epidural haematomas and tumours. This should be considered a surgical emergency, requiring urgent investigation with MRI and management with surgical intervention or radiotherapy.

Clinical features

- Presentation is usually of acute pain, preceded by a history of chronic pain of varying intensity. Cauda equina syndrome should be considered with a history of urinary retention, faecal incontinence and saddle anaesthesia.

- A triggering event is often not identified but a prior history of lifting or sports activity may be reported.

- Pain usually occurs in a dermatomal distribution, depending on the nerve root involved, and radiates down the leg – described as an ache, burning sensation or shooting pain.

- Dermatomal symptoms include the following.
  - *L4 nerve root involvement* – pain and sensory changes in the anterior and medial aspect of the thigh and calf.

- *L5 nerve root involvement* – pain and sensory changes in the lateral aspect of the thigh and anterior shin.
- *S1 nerve root involvement* – calf pain and major source of pain and sensory changes in the lateral border and plantar surface of the foot.
- Associated perineal parasthesia suggests cauda equina syndrome.
- Neurological examination may be normal in disc prolapse, but abnormal gait and subtle muscle weakness may be demonstrated; however, the latter may be confounded by limitation secondary to pain.
- Additional tests include the following.
  - *Straight-leg raise test* – pain secondary to 'sciatica', resulting in reduction in passive hip flexion, with the knee extended, on the affected side.
  - *Lasegue's test* – foot dorsiflexion worsening sciatic pain.
  - *The bow-string test* – stretch the nerve roots (hip at 90°, knee at 90°) by pressing centrally in the popliteal fossa, to delineate between tight hamstrings and neural inflammation/compression.
- With cauda equina syndrome, sensory abnormality, muscle weakness and wasting, poor anal tone and signs of urinary retention may be demonstrated.

Radiological features

MRI
- The imaging modality of choice. If this is contraindicated, CT (myelography) can be helpful.
- If there is a preceding history of trauma, plain radiographs and/or CT should be performed to rule out fractures as a cause of the symptoms.

Features
- On T2-weighted imaging, low-signal disc material is seen protruding into the central canal, with effacement of the high-signal CSF around the nerve roots.
- Identification of nerve root compression, or irritation, is best seen on the axial images using both T1- and T2-weighted sequences (Fig. 48.1).
- Exiting neural foramina should contain high-signal fat wrapping around the low-signal exiting nerve root. Effacement or obliteration of this fat signal by low-signal disc material suggests distortion or compression of the nerve root. Although this can be seen on axial images, sagittal sequences help to confirm these findings.
- It is important to have a good grasp of the anatomical relationship of the nerve roots to disc herniation. For example at L4/5, the L4 nerve roots exit at the neural foraminae, while the L5 nerve roots traverse the lateral recess of the canal.
- A sequestered disc is one that has separated from the main disc, resulting in a 'free' fragment lying within the canal. It is important to recognize this, as it may cause nerve root compression in an atypical dermatomal distribution. Surgeons should be made aware of this finding as the surgical approach will be altered as a result.

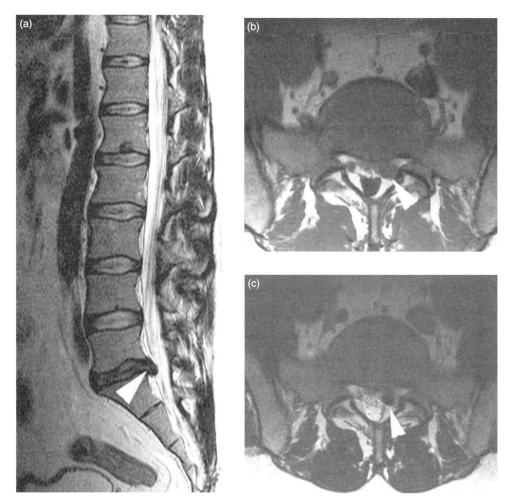

Fig. 48.1. (a) Sagittal T2W MRI demonstrating left paracentral disc protrusion at L5/S1 (arrowhead). Axial (b) T1W and (c) T2W MRI images confirming the left paracentral disc protrusion, causing compression of the left traversing S1 nerve root in the lateral recess (arrowhead).

Chapter

49

Deep vein thrombosis

Characteristics

- Imbalance in Virchow's triad of venous stasis, injury to the vascular wall, and a hypercoagulable state leads to venous thrombosis.

- Lower-extremity deep vein thrombosis (DVT) occurs most commonly, with an incidence of 1 per 1,000 population. The incidence in hospitalized patients is considerably higher and varies from 20% to 70%.

- Risk factors include immobilization >3 days, pregnancy and postpartum states, major surgery in the previous 4 weeks (particularly orthopaedic), long-haul flights (>4 hours), cancer, previous DVT, multiple burns or trauma, vasculitides, haematological disorders leading to prothrombotic states, intravenous drug abuse and the oral contraceptive pill.

- The thrombus may fragment or dislodge, leading to pulmonary embolism.

- Post-thrombotic syndrome occurs in 15% of patients, presenting with pain, oedema, venous claudication, skin pigmentation, dermatitis and ulceration.

- The *Wells score* (see Appendix VII) is a clinical prediction guide for DVT, incorporating risk factors, signs and possible alternative diagnoses, thus allowing physicians to assess a patient's risk.

Clinical features

- The severity and extent of symptoms are related to the degree of venous obstruction and vessel wall inflammation. However, patients may be asymptomatic, with no specific symptoms or findings to suggest the diagnosis.

- Common symptoms include unilateral limb or calf pain and swelling. Symptoms of pulmonary embolism may also be reported.

- Examination may reveal unilateral oedema, with tenderness localized to the calf muscles and along the deep veins, over the medial aspect of the thigh.

- Beware of superficial thrombophlebitis, an alternative diagnosis that can also occur in conjunction with a DVT.

- *Homan's sign* is present in approximately one-third of patients with DVT and represents discomfort in the calf on passive dorsiflexion of the foot.

- *Phlegmasia cerulea dolens* describes the reddish purple discoloration secondary to venous engorgement and obstruction.

Radiological features

Ultrasound

- The imaging modality of choice for the diagnosis of deep vein thrombosis. Increasingly used in emergency departments by non-radiologists as a point-of-care bedside test.

Features (Fig. 49.1)

- Venous compression is performed from the common femoral vein to the level of the trifurcation of the popliteal vein. Colour Doppler and spectral Doppler can be used to assess flow within the vein. Augmentation can help to demonstrate flow by squeezing the calf while using Doppler imaging. Assessment of calf veins can be performed depending on local policies and expertise.

- Thrombus appears echogenic within a normally anechoic lumen. However, acute thrombus can appear anechoic, and the diagnosis therefore relies on the identification of a distended and non-compressible vein, with reduced/absent Doppler flow.

- The proximal extent of the thrombus should be identified where possible, as involvement of the iliac vessels or the inferior vena cava increases the risk of pulmonary embolism.

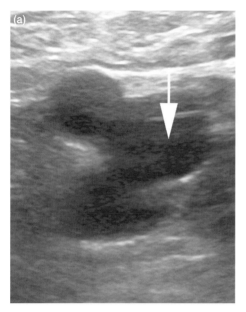
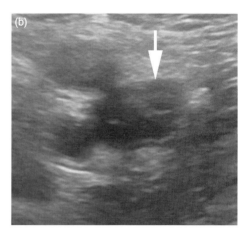
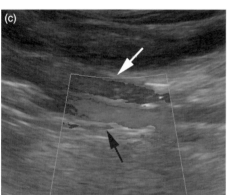
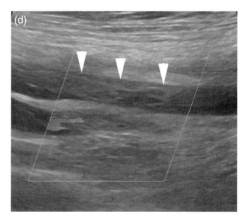

Fig. 49.1. (a) Transverse ultrasound image demonstrates normal appearance of the femoral vein (arrow) and (b) echogenic thrombus within the femoral vein (arrow) (c) Duplex ultrasound image demonstrating normal flow within the femoral vein (white arrow) and superficial femoral artery (black arrow). (d) Duplex ultrasound image demonstrating echogenic thrombus within the femoral vein (arrowheads) with absence of colour flow on Doppler.

Appendix I ABCD^2 scoring system

- Used to help assess the risk of early stroke following a transient ischaemic attack (TIA).
- The score is calculated according to five important clinical features:

A – Age	>60 years	1 point
B – Blood pressure at presentation	≥140/90 mmHg	1 point
C – Clinical features	Unilateral weakness	2 points
	Speech disturbance without weakness	1 point
D – Duration of symptoms	≥60 minutes	2 points
	10–59 minutes	1 point
D – Diabetes	Present	1 point

- The subsequent risk for stroke within the first 2 days following a TIA is:

ABCD^2 score	Risk of stroke at 2 days
0–3	1%
4–5	4%
6–7	8%

Further reading

Johnston, S. C., Rothwell, P. M., Nguyen-Huynh, M. N., Giles, M. F., Elkins, J. S., Bernstein, A. L., Sidney, S. (2007). Validation and refinement of scores to predict very early stroke risk after transient ischaemic attack. *Lancet* **369**, 283–92.

Appendix II Proposed algorithm for the emergency management of acute stroke

- Active management in the initial hours after stroke aims to preserve the ischaemic brain from infarction.
- For recognition of suspected stroke, use the FAST test:

F – Facial movements	New asymmetry
A – Arm movements	Unilateral arm weakness
S – Speech	Dysarthria or aphasia
T – Telephone 999 in the community	Bleep acute stroke team if symptoms present

Initial management

- Instigate resuscitative measures according to ABC assessment.
- If conscious, the patient should sit up.
- Nil by mouth.
- Oxygen to maintain saturation >95%.
- 100 ml 10% dextrose i.v. if blood glucose <3 mmol/l.
- Intravenous saline if hypotensive.
- Blood pressure should only be lowered in the acute phase if hypertension is likely to lead to complications (e.g. hypertensive encephalopathy, aortic aneurysm).
- Baseline investigations including ECG and blood tests.
- Assess risk of aspiration, using a validated swallowing screening tool.
- Transfer to an Acute Stroke Unit.

Urgent CT imaging (or MRI where available) of the head should take place for the following patients

- Anticoagulant therapy (e.g. warfarin).
- Coagulopathies.
- Depressed level of consciousness.
- Papilloedema.
- Neck stiffness.
- Severe headache.
- Progressive or fluctuating neurological symptoms.
- If neurological deficit persists on arrival to hospital, and the onset of symptoms was within 3 hours, thrombolytic therapy may be considered. The current UK licence is for

treatment of patients between 18 and 80 years and within 3 hours of the onset of symptoms.

- CT (or MRI) must be performed prior to thrombolysis to exclude cerebral haemorrhage.

Exclusion criteria for thrombolytic therapy for acute stroke

- No clear time of symptom onset.
- Decreased level of consciousness.
- Very severe stroke (e.g. NIH Stroke Scale score >25).
- Mild clinical deficit or rapidly resolving symptoms.
- Seizure at stroke onset.
- Symptoms suggestive of subarachnoid haemorrhage (SAH), even if the CT is normal.
- CT demonstrates any intracranial haemorrhage.
- CT scan showing hypodensity of an evolving infarction >1/3 of arterial territory, oedema or midline shift.
- CNS tumour, aneurysm or arteriovenous malformation (AVM).
- BP >185/110 after two attempts to reduce blood pressure.
- Glucose <2.7 mmol/l or >22.2 mmol/l.
- INR >1.4, APTT >40, or platelet count <100,000 mm^3.
- Ischaemic stroke, serious head injury, or neurosurgery within the last 3 months.
- Past history of intracranial haemorrhage.
- Pregnancy.
- Standard contraindications for thrombolysis applied to myocardial infarction.

Thrombolysis protocol

- Administer Alteplase 0.9 mg × body weight in kg (maximum 90 mg).
- Give 10% of total dose as a bolus over 2 minutes at 1 mg/ml.
- Infuse 90% of total dose at 1 mg/ml over 60 minutes.

Post-thrombolysis protocol

- Assess GCS and perform standard neurological observations hourly for the first 12 hours, and then every 2 hours for the next 12 hours.
- BP and pulse every 15 minutes for 2 hours, then every 30 minutes for 6 hours, then hourly for 16 hours.
- Treat BP greater than 185/110.
- Repeat head CT at 24 hours, or sooner if neurological deterioration occurs.
- Avoid heparin and antiplatelet agents (including aspirin) until repeat CT at 24 hours has excluded haemorrhage.
- Avoid i.m. injections or unnecessary venous or arterial punctures.
- If clinically significant bleeding occurs, stop the thrombolytic therapy, perform urgent CT scan, and give cryoprecipitate (discuss with Haematology).
- Give supportive i.v. fluids as necessary.

Appendix III Glasgow coma scale

- The most widely used scoring system for quantifying level of consciousness following traumatic brain injury.
- Coma is defined as a score <8.

Glasgow coma scale for adults

Eye opening	Verbal response	Motor response
1 – None	1 – None	1 – None
2 – To pain	2 – Incomprehensible sound	2 – Extension to pain
3 – To speech	3 – Inappropriate words	3 – Abnormal flexion to pain
4 – Spontaneous	4 – Confused/disorientated	4 – Withdraws from pain
	5 – Orientated	5 – Localizes to pain
		6 – Obeys command

Adapted Glasgow coma scale for children

Eye opening	Verbal response	Motor response
1 – None	1 – None	1 – None
2 – To pain	2 – Inconsolable, agitated	2 – Extension to pain
3 – To speech	3 – Inconsistently inconsolable, moaning	3 – Abnormal flexion to pain
4 – Spontaneous	4 – Cries but consolable, inappropriate interaction	4 – Withdraws from pain
	5 – Smiles, orientated to sounds, follows objects, interacts	5 – Withdraws from touch
		6 – Moves spontaneously or purposefully

Further reading

Teasdale, G., Jennett, B. (1974). Assessment of coma and impaired consciousness: a practical scale. *Lancet* **13**, 81–4.

Appendix IV Adapted NICE guideline for CT scanning in adult head injury

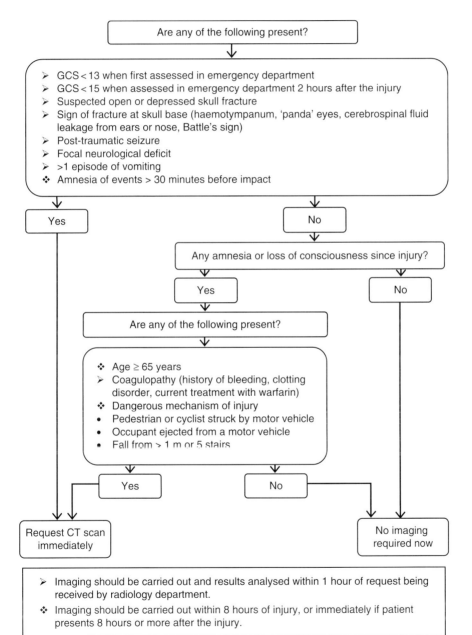

Are any of the following present?

- ➤ GCS < 13 when first assessed in emergency department
- ➤ GCS < 15 when assessed in emergency department 2 hours after the injury
- ➤ Suspected open or depressed skull fracture
- ➤ Sign of fracture at skull base (haemotympanum, 'panda' eyes, cerebrospinal fluid leakage from ears or nose, Battle's sign)
- ➤ Post-traumatic seizure
- ➤ Focal neurological deficit
- ➤ >1 episode of vomiting
- ❖ Amnesia of events > 30 minutes before impact

Yes

No

Any amnesia or loss of consciousness since injury?

Yes

No

Are any of the following present?

- ❖ Age ≥ 65 years
- ➤ Coagulopathy (history of bleeding, clotting disorder, current treatment with warfarin)
- ❖ Dangerous mechanism of injury
- • Pedestrian or cyclist struck by motor vehicle
- • Occupant ejected from a motor vehicle
- • Fall from > 1 m or 5 stairs

Yes

No

Request CT scan immediately

No imaging required now

- ➤ Imaging should be carried out and results analysed within 1 hour of request being received by radiology department.
- ❖ Imaging should be carried out within 8 hours of injury, or immediately if patient presents 8 hours or more after the injury.

Appendix V Adapted NICE guideline for CT scanning in children (<16 years old) head injury

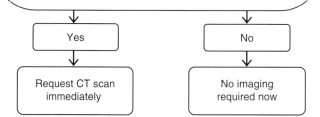

Are any of the following present?

- Witnessed loss of consciousness lasting > 5 minutes
- Amnesia (antegrade or retrograde) lasting > 5 minutes
- Abnormal drowsiness
- 3 or more discrete episodes of vomiting
- Clinical suspicious of non-accidental injury
- Post traumatic seizure but no history of epilepsy
- Age > 1 year. GCS < 14 on assessment in the emergency department
- Age < 1 year. GCS (paediatric) < 15 on assessment in the emergency department
- Suspicion of open or depressed skull injury or tense fontanelle
- Any sign of basal skull fracture (haemotympanum, 'panda' eyes, cerebrospinal fluid leakage from ears or nose, Battle's sign)
- Focal neurological deficit
- Age < 1 year: presence of bruise, swelling or laceration > 5 cm on the head
- Dangerous mechanism of injury (high-speed road traffic accident either as pedestrian, cyclist or vehicle occupant, fall from > 3 m, high-speed injury from a projectile or an object)

Yes → Request CT scan immediately

No → No imaging required now

Appendix VI Information required prior to neurosurgical referral

- Before contacting the neurosurgeon, vital information and an updated clinical evaluation must be collated.
- The following list includes the minimum details that must be immediately available:
  - Referring hospital and named consultant
  - Patient demographics with hospital number
  - Date and time of incident
  - Time of admission
  - History of event
  - Physiological observations

Time	HR	BP	RR	O₂sat	GCS Eyes	GCS Speech	GCS Motor	Right pupil reacts	Right pupil size	Left pupil reacts	Left pupil size
On arrival											
On transfer											

  - CT scan(s) at referring hospital Yes/No
  - Result of CT scan of head
  - CT scan of neck/chest/abdomen/pelvis/face
  - Other injuries
  - Relevant past medical history
  - Allergies
  - Drug history
  - Last ingestion
  - Interventions:

Airway:	Guedel	ETT
Breathing:	Spontaneous	IPPV
Circulation:	Fluids Urinary	catheter

  - Drugs given
  - Tetanus
  - Blood test results

- ○ Cross-match
- ○ Arterial blood gas
- ○ Urinalysis
- ○ Next of kin contact details: Notified Yes/No
- ○ Medical escort

Appendix VII Wells scores for deep vein thrombosis and pulmonary embolism

- Clinical prediction rules which are commonly used in everyday clinical practice.

Wells score for deep vein thrombosis (DVT)

Active cancer	+1 point
Bedridden recently >3 days or major surgery within 4 weeks	+1 point
Calf swelling >3 cm compared with the other leg	+1 point
Collateral (non-varicose) superficial veins present	+1 point
Entire leg swollen	+1 point
Localized tenderness along the deep venous system	+1 point
Pitting oedema, greater in the symptomatic leg	+1 point
Paralysis, paresis, or recent plaster immobilization of the lower extremity	+1 point
Previously documented DVT	+1 point
Alternative diagnosis to DVT as likely or more likely	−2 points

- Score ≥2 – suggests high risk of DVT, and imaging of leg veins is recommended.
- Score <2 – DVT is unlikely. Consider blood test such as D-dimer to rule out DVT.

Modified Wells score for pulmonary embolism (PE)

Clinical signs and symptoms of DVT	+3 points
PE is number 1 diagnosis, or equally likely	+3 points
Heart rate >100 bpm	+1.5 points
Immobilization at least 3 days, or surgery in the previous 4 weeks	+1.5 points
Previous objectively diagnosed PE or DVT	+1.5 points
Haemoptysis	+1 point
Malignancy with treatment within 6 months, or on palliative treatment	+1 point

- Score >4 – PE likely. Consider diagnostic imaging.
- Score ≤4 – PE unlikely. Consider blood test such as D-dimer to rule out PE.

Index